AF560017

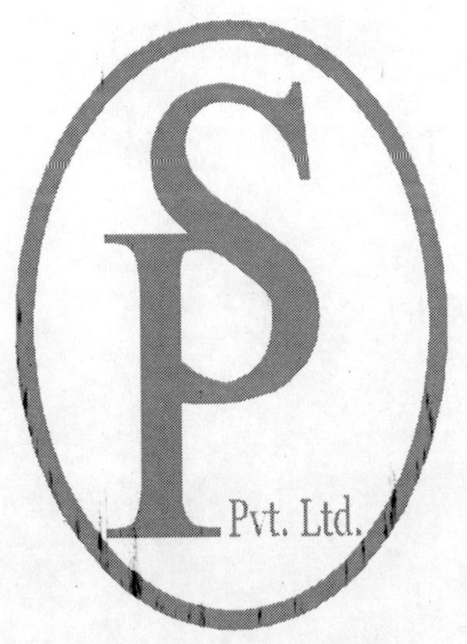
SP
Pvt. Ltd.

Under-Nutrition and Vulnerability

Moumita Mukherjee
Development Economist & Research Director
Thematic Action Research Analytics (TARA) Foundation
20, Bireswar Chatterjee Street, Swapnapuran,
Bally, Howrah – 711 201

2018

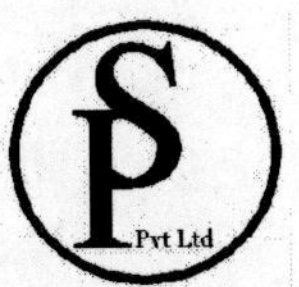

Studium Press (India) Pvt. Ltd.

Under-Nutrition and Vulnerability

ISBN: 978-93-85046-19-3

Published by:

Studium Press (India) Pvt. Ltd.
4735/22, 2nd Floor, Prakash Deep Building
(Near Delhi Medical Association),
Ansari Road, Darya Ganj, New Delhi-110 002
Tel.: + 91-11-43240200-15 (15 lines); Fax: 91-11-43240215
E-mail: studiumpress@gmail.com

Printed at India

About the Author

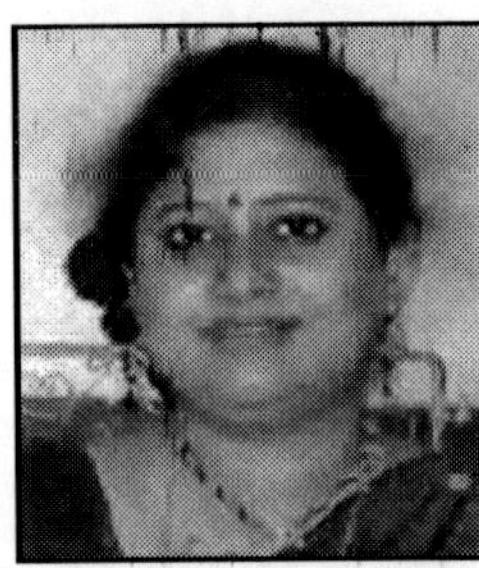

Dr. Moumita Mukherjee possesses experience in social research for last 10 years related to poverty, livelihood, health, nutrition, water and sanitation, education and child protection. She works in international and national projects in UNICEF, IIHMR, CTS, Sigma Research, and IDSK. She has 12 national and international publications. Her research interests are multi-dimensional vulnerability, social inequity, financial catastrophe, climatic change, social poverty, malnutrition, violence against women and children, healthcare and health seeking behaviour, accessibility to health and educational services, water-sanitation and hygiene, rural livelihood and institutional mainstreaming.

Acknowledgement

I express my gratitude to Sir Ratan Tata Trust Fellowship awarded by Institute for Social and Economic Change Bangalore. I am grateful to vulnerable communities in my study area who spent their valuable time to help my research.

I dedicate this work to my family (*my daughter, my father and my husband*) because without their support I would never achieve any goal in my life.

Moumita Mukherjee

Preface

Childhood under-nutrition is a curse on the developing world leaving the children to achieve sub-optimal equilibrium with respect to one non-income dimension of well being. Sub-optimal because, production of health capital is inadequate due to lack of supply of nutrition inputs required to produce healthy children. Though there is substantial economic growth and poverty reduction in Indian economy, how far such scenario can be sustained in future becomes questionable after considering little achievement in health and nutrition of the vulnerable child population in the country. Since, if their health and nutritional achievements remain behind then there is a possibility to have negative impact on the economy in the long run. Children's health outcomes are highly associated with their nutritional status. Nutritional status affects physical and cognitive development and therefore influences future productive capacity of individual. Thus, nutritional achievements control the future earning potential. Again, it is also true that poor and contextually vulnerable children are more malnourished. Literatures name it feedback loop of poverty and malnutrition.

So, different development agencies and donor organizations are now concern about the fact that may be the mainstreaming of nutritional interventions in poverty reduction strategies will be helpful to sustain economic development. In this background my work will try to explore whether the transformation in thought process from poverty to vulnerability can throw new light on the determinants of malnutrition after assessing the link between changing profile of malnutrition and poverty and inequity in India. It is expected to help the research community to understand the pathway through which better health and nutrition of children can be assured.

Moumita Mukherjee

Table of Contents

1

Poverty, Vulnerability and Under-Nutrition: An Overview of the Trajectories

Poverty is a chronic ailment in our socio-economy. It increases the burden of deprivation, reduces capability to earn living, and raises the impact of any external shock manifold. Poor population is under continuous threat of any disease – whether it is being social, psychosocial or physiological. They remain always at risk of several social, economic, environmental, biological, spatial uncertainties so that the future becomes susceptible to any change, any dynamics. Sub-optimal capabilities limit the attainment of every dimension of well-being and surrounding context accelerates the deterioration further – leading to poverty deepening. Poverty trajectory or the history of its pattern reflects a clear nexus with different risks and vulnerabilities preceding as well as following it. Literatures developed the concepts of poverty and vulnerability – both from broader as well as narrower perspectives. Many of them generalized the concepts deep inside the theories whereas, many works provide empirical connotation. Some of the previous research works provide generalizations with particular issues and some of them discuss more than one. Empirical works also follow the analogous mode.

Multiple concepts of poverty and ever increasing multidimensional issues gradually developed the concept of vulnerability thinking deeper into poverty in dynamic sense through probabilistic lens. Concept of relative poverty against absolute poverty evidences the existence of inequalities within economies (in macro sense), communities or households (in micro sense) in several welfare dimensions (Sen, 1987, Linnermayr *et al.,* 2008). However, such ex post measures *i.e.*, the phenomena which already actually felt compared to ex ante measures (phenomena which are anticipated and measured in probabilistic way) are limited in power in the sense that they fail to predict the future of the socio-economy. In other words, if a current situation depicts rapid economic growth accompanied by poverty reduction, how far such growth is inclusive and poverty is distribution corrected can be measured. But whether in medium or longer run this rate of growth and poverty reduction can be sustained or in what degree is difficult to predict. Similarly for economies facing diminishing return to factors of production *e.g.* labour, how far the scenario is related to inclusive growth or inclusive development can be estimated but in the similar manner whether ex ante poverty and/ or inequality will affect future labor productivity, its complex pathways through elements of economic development and related dynamics will remain unexplored with traditional concepts of poverty and inequality. Here vulnerability to poverty and inequality evolves with its immense significance to sustain economic development and accelerate the pace of economic growth.

Though a large number of literatures are available on vulnerability to poor health, poverty, climate change, disaster and so on in isolated manner; multidimensional vulnerability calls for attention followed by action. Literatures views vulnerability as an ex ante concept. It is the likelihood of experiencing loss in the future relative to some benchmark of welfare (may be poverty line) caused by uncertainties like climatic events, disease outbreaks, price shocks or market failures. The degree of vulnerability depends on the characteristics, frequency and magnitude of the risk as well as causal relation with household's ability to respond to the risk given its entitlement bundle. Literatures evidence temporal variation of vulnerability; poor and near-poor showing average monotone sequence due to limited access to entitlements and institutions (broadly defined) leading to higher perceived opportunity cost, weak coping strategies and supply side ineffectiveness or less effectiveness (Alwang *et al.,* 2001; Elbers and Gunning, 2003; Ligon and Schechter, 2003; Calvo and Dercon, 2005; Baeza and Packard, 2006; Azam and Imai, 2009).

CONTEXT OF UNDER-NUTRITION

Child under-nutrition is a curse on the developing world children. It implies physical and cognitive growth deceleration that occurs as a response to suboptimal nutrition to maintain equilibrium between genetic growth potential and nutritional intake. In other words, sub-optimal because, production of health capital is inadequate due to lack of supply of nutrition inputs required for producing healthy children (Smith and Haddad, 1999). Though there occurred a substantial economic growth and poverty reduction in the Indian economy, how far such scenario is sufficient to bring better health of child population is questionable (IIPS, 2007). Since, if their health and nutritional achievements remain behind then there is a possibility to have negative impact on the economy in the long run since nutritional status affects future productive capacity of individual through physical and cognitive development and thereby control the future earning potential (Dasgupta and Roy, 1986; Mahal *et al.,* 2001; Linnermayr *et al.,* 2008). Existing literature establishes poor children are more undernourished (Navaneetham and Jose, 2005). Literatures name this two way relationship as feedback loop of poverty and under-nutrition (Deolalikar, 2004; Svedberg, 2000; Navaneetham and Jose, 2005; Hong and Mishra, 2006; Svedberg, 2008). However, different development agencies and donor organizations are concerned about mainstreaming nutritional interventions in poverty reduction strategies to sustain economic development which is needed to be properly targeted (Shekar and Lee, 2006). Human well-being and development is under a threat with millions of children under the age of five are malnourished, more specifically undernourished.

Under-nutrition implying chronic or acute protein and energy deficiency *i.e.,* macronutrient deficiency as well as vitamin and mineral deficiency *i.e.,* micronutrient deficiency - is responsible for 2.2 million deaths and 21 percent disability adjusted life years among children under the age of five in low and middle income countries (Black *et al.,* 2008).

As indicated in Figure 1.1, chronic childhood under-nutrition in India declined by nine percentage points in a period of fifteen years while, income poverty was reduced by eighteen percentage points (IIPS, 2007; Human Development Report, 2001). In this background my work will try to find why in spite of fall in absolute poverty, childhood under-nutrition – one non-income indicator of well-being - has not been reduced sufficiently in India.

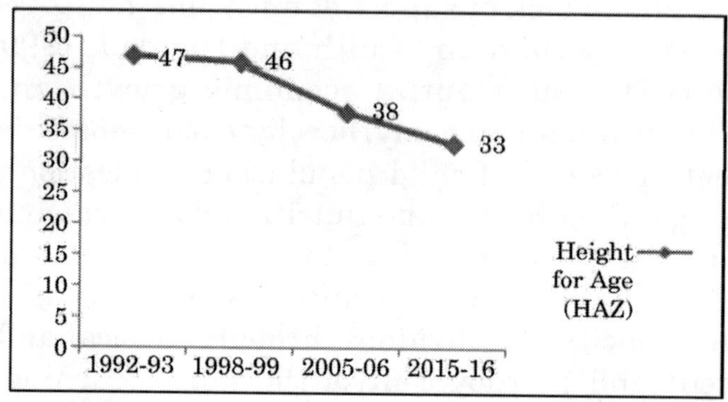

Figure 1.1: Percentage of malnourished children in India in three time points (1992-93, 1998-99, 2005-06, 2015-16)

The World Scenario in Relation to Chronic Under-Nutrition

Long-term deficiencies in nutritional status are indicated by stunting. Underweight or wasting indicates mainly the acute under-nutrition *i.e.* short-term deficiencies. In the present work I investigate chronic or long-term under-nutrition instead of acute under-nutrition. This is because of two vital reasons. Acute under-nutrition masks the chronic deficiencies (UNICEF, 2009). Another reason is, economic status impacts the nutritional status of children slowly through a longer period of time. So such impact is better captured in chronic nutritional deficiencies rather than acute nutritional deficiencies (Poel *et al.*, 2008). Stunting more accurately reflects nutritional deficiencies and illness that occur during the most critical periods of growth and development in the early years of life (UNICEF, 2009). Recent estimates of UNICEF (2009) show that the global burden of stunting is much higher than that of underweight. The number of stunted children under five years of age is 200 million whereas the number of underweight children under same population subgroup is 130 million in the developing world (ibid.). A few studies use chronic under-nutrition as poverty indicator (Radhakrishna *et al.*, 2006). UNICEF study argues that Government, donors and global partners who use underweight as an indicator are overlooking a great persisting problem of under-nutrition which is damaging the society over a longer period of time. This huge burden should be an issue of great concern. It is also difficult to achieve some other goals under Millennium Development Goals if the first goal is not accomplished (UNICEF, 2009). So the need of the hour is exploring the crucial contributors to chronic under-nutrition (or in other words stunting) and controlling them through cost-effective interventions.

Current World Situation

Twenty four countries are burdened with 80 percent of world's childhood stunting and more than 90 percent of developing world's stunted children live in Asia and Africa (Table 1.1).

Among low and middle-income countries, India shares the greatest burden of stunted children (31%) compared to any other. Among other high, medium or low prevalent countries, each of them shares less than 10 percent of total prevalence of developing world.

More than one third of child deaths are due to child and mother's undernourishment. Thirty seven percent of neonatal

Table 1.1: Prevalence of chronic under-nutrition, number of chronically undernourished children and country's share of prevalence of stunting in different developing countries in total developing world

Country	*Prevalence of Chronic under-nutrition (in per 100)*	*Number of children who are stunted (thousands, 2008)*	*% in developing world total (195.1 million)*
India	48	60,788	31.2%
China	15	12,685	6.5%
Nigeria	41	10,158	5.2%
Pakistan	42	9,868	5.1%
Indonesia	37	7,688	3.9%
Bangladesh	43	7,219	3.7%
Ethiopia	51	6,768	3.5%
Democratic Republic of the Congo	46	5,382	2.8%
Philippines	34	3,617	1.9%
United Republic of Tanzania	44	3,359	1.7%
Afghanistan	59	2,910	1.5%
Egypt	29	2,730	1.4%
Vietnam	36	2,619	1.3%
Uganda	38	2,355	1.2%
Sudan	40	2,305	1.2%
Kenya	35	2,269	1.2%
Yemen	58	2,154	1.1%
Myanmar	41	1,880	1.0%
Nepal	49	1,743	<1%
Mozambique	44	1,670	<1%
Madagascar	53	1,622	<1%
Mexico	16	1,594	<1%
Niger	47	1,473	<1%
South Africa	27	1,425	<1%

Source: UNICEF, 2009

death is directly related to under-nutrition. Fifty percent of child deaths from different diseases like Acute Respiratory Infection, Diarrhoea, Malaria, Measles, and HIV/AIDs are indirectly related to under-nutrition (Caulfield *et al.,* 2004).

Among ten developing countries that contribute most of the chronic under-nutrition burden, five of them are in Asia. These countries are India, Bangladesh, Indonesia, Pakistan and Philippines. South Asia is the hub of the most undernourished. Though India does not have the highest prevalence of stunted children, it has the greatest number of stunted children. India thus accounts for more than three out of every ten stunted children in the developing world.

STATUS OF STUNTING IN DEVELOPING COUNTRIES

In developing world, during last one and half decade stunting has decreased by 11 percentage points on average (Table 1.1). In Asia it declined from 44 percent to 30 percent and in Africa overall the fall is from 38 percent to 34 percent (UNICEF, 2009). South American countries like Bolivia and South and East Asian countries like Bangladesh, Vietnam, and China had shown more than 20 percent decline in stunting during this decade (UNICEF, 2009). National Family Health Survey data shows that, stunting prevalence among children under the age of three in India has declined from 47 percent to 38 percent in one and half decade (IIPS, 2007).

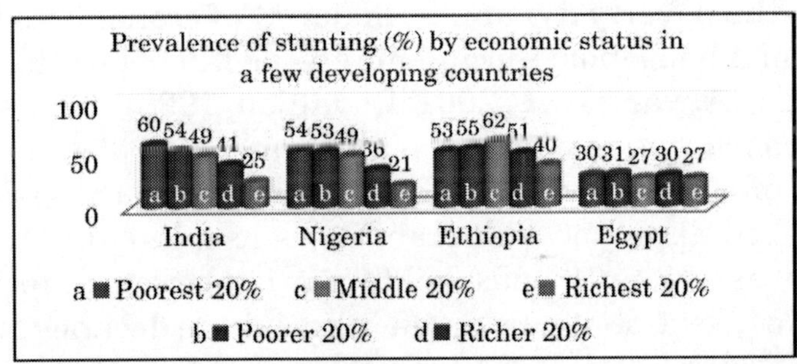

Figure 1.2: Inequality in nutritional status by economic quintile (*Source*: UNICEF, 2009)

It has long been established that in India stunting is higher among the poor (which is not true for all the developing countries) (*e.g.*, Figure 1.2). Though poverty is considered as basic determinant of stunting and in last two decades India experienced a substantial decline in incidence of poverty (as per the evidence from Human Development Report, 2001), the prevalence of stunting remained more or less stagnant. Then the question remains- why in spite of considerable amount of poverty reduction, there is little decline in chronic under-nutrition prevalence during the last two decades. So, in this book I will explore deep inside the ex ante poverty and its influence on under-nutrition to assess how far it is responsible for the said diminishing return. Next, I will review the existing literature on this issue to build the foundation of my research.

SOURCES OF VULNERABILITY

Theoretical and empirical studies broadly categorize the sources of vulnerabilities into – 1) Economic, 2) Social and political, 3) Disaster related, 4) Demographic, 5) Geographic, 6) Climate related, 7) Health related, and so on or interaction of some or many of them.

Economic Vulnerability

According to *Economics* literature, the term vulnerability is implicit in the poverty dynamics; majority of economists focus on likelihood of a household's economic status fall below the poverty line in future (Alwang *et al.*, 2001; Ravallion, 1998). They estimate *income* or *consumption* dispersion as the measure of vulnerability – outcome of a process of household responses to the risk (ibid.). In *asset* based approach vulnerability is associated with loss or depletion of assets. Such households may not be consumption poor but they are investment poor as their asset base declines over time and are unable or less able to generate surplus to protect, maintain or enhance their assets (Reaedon and Vosti, 1995). As asset based approach is more stable measure with respect to temporal aspect, considering asset inequality and related ex ante possibilities able to bring sustainable policy suggestions. The investment poverty concept is forward looking and dynamic (Alwang *et al.,* 2001). Vulnerability as concept in *livelihood* literature is defined as the probability that livelihood stress will occur, implying the probability of that household to be deficient in means for mitigating or coping risk without incurring loss after idiosyncratic or covariate shock (Chambers, 1989; Mukherjee, 2014). Vulnerability in *food security* literature is defined as the collective effects of risk and of the ability of an individual or household to *cope* with those risks and to recover from a shock or deterioration of current status(Maxwell *et al.,* 2000; Mukherjee, 2014).

In India, poverty, under-nutrition linkage is generating vulnerability through recurrent entrapment within under-nutrition morbidity vicious circle which lessens the ability to engage in productive and remunerative employment (Heller and Drake, 1979; Gaiha *et al.,* 2014). Worse socioeconomic status leads to trap people in debt and related insecurities put them to select insecure livelihoods like sex trade (Reed *et al.,* 2010). According to one detailed research on impact of macroeconomic crisis on nutritional achievement of children substantiates that financial crisis at macro level reduces price of agricultural product and access to credit in the market leading to reduction of agricultural production. Along with these factors, low employment and volatility of food prices reduced the demand. Therefore decline in food consumption and expenditure on health preceded by fluctuation in income increased the vulnerability to worse nutritional and health status of children. Different earlier works discussed their theoretical and empirical works on how under-nutrition at early stages in life increases economic vulnerability to poverty at later stages *via* labour productivity (Basta *et al.,* 1979; Dasgupta and Ray, 1986, 1987; Strauss and Thomas, 1998; Jayachandran and Pandey, 2012). In works of Imai and other economists (2013), engagement in rural non-farm economy reduces poverty and vulnerability in India among average educated and nourished people and put them into virtuous circle. Authors suggest skill training, microfinance initiatives would be helpful to encourage diversification.But to sustain such initiatives in the longer run, reduction of under-nutrition and reducing the barriers towards nourished development of children are need of the hour to break the under-nutrition vulnerability vicious circle.

Social Vulnerability

But vulnerability is a broader concept encompassing not only any uni- dimensional volatility, but also includes risks related to educational attainment, gender, health, domestic violence, crime and/or social exclusion (Coudouel and Hentschel, 2000). Where it takes into account the degree of resilience, sensitivity along with susceptibility with respect to all the above mentioned facets. *Sociologists* use the term "vulnerability" to capture the dimensions of poverty which are not captured by money-metric measures or asset based measures. They work on vulnerabilities with respect to capabilities, deprivation or exclusion to determine the process of being poor considering developmental aspects (Moser and Holland, 1997; Bebbington, 1999). As found in different literatures, socio-structural rigidities and inequalities perpetuate difficulties and shape the coping ability curve to have a continuous declining trend (Devereux *et al.,* 2006).

Literatures on social vulnerability depict presence of poverty as well as higher prevalence of under-nutrition among lower social strata (IIPS, 2007; Himanshu and Stern, 2011). Thus vicious circle of poverty and under-nutrition put them into socioeconomic vulnerabilities in the long-run (Mukherjee, 2014). Furthermore, less acceptability of institutional care in health and nutrition causes intergenerational transfer of under-nutrition creating the trajectory of future vulnerabilities through reduction of health capital (IIHMR, 2010).

Disaster Related Vulnerability

In *disaster management* literature, degrees of vulnerabilities in households, communities etc., include risk of experiencing natural disaster and responsiveness to those risks (Blackie *et al.,* 1994).

According to their definition of vulnerability "...characteristics of a person or group in terms of their capacity to anticipate, cope with, resist, and recover from the impact of a natural disaster" (Blackie *et al.,* 1994; p. 9).

With respect to Indian subcontinent, there exists different coastal areas, semi-urban areas or urban locale suffering from vulnerability spirals and needs convergence in research of multi-hazards and long-term assessment of risks and resilience. One similar study on coastal area of Odisha found that vulnerability dynamics between big or smaller repetitive climatic shocks, lack of alternative livelihoods and limited or no institutional involvement weakens the resilience (Chhotray and Few, 2012). According to the study inference, NGO activity and the State actions are complementary to each other and both are required to foster resilience in needy affected areas (ibid.). Anecdotally, also in Odisha evidences suggest association between long-term under-nutrition among children who are exposed to flood at their early years of life and long-term flood prevention programmes are recommended to prevent children from under-nutrition.

Vulnerabilities Related to Demography

From *Demography* literature, evidences show that households headed by women, children or elderly are more vulnerable as they are constrained by the amount of their productive capacity (Devereux *et al.,* 2006). Such constraints are either structurally determined or influenced by poor health status (ibid.). If a young male earning member becomes chronically ill or suffers from an accident which obstructs from doing harder manual labour, that family becomes vulnerable and the vulnerability increases cumulatively as the process of becoming a woman-, elderly- or child-headed household starts and continues (ibid.). One study on India, Bangladesh and Nepal exploring the impact of existence of siblings on childhood under-nutrition revealed son preference/daughter aversion affects childhood nutritional status in South Asia (Raj *et al.,* 2015). It is evident from there is that, having brothers worsens girl risk for acute under-nutrition (wasting), where having multiple sisters raises girl risk for chronic under-nutrition (stunting) whereas boy under-nutrition rates are less affected by siblings. Another study in Mali, Africa explored the impact of climate change on under-nutrition and evidenced that gradual changing trend in climate along with demographic and livelihood trends are likely to increase the vulnerabilities to under-nutrition and related outcomes (Marta *et al.,* 2012).

Geographic Vulnerabilities

Geographic adversities create vulnerabilities to future poverty through limiting the physical access to market transactions – whether it is related to supply or demand, selling of products to earn or seeking food and non-food items for consumption (Jordon *et al.*, 2004; Peters *et al.*, 2008). Regional variation in access to health and nutrition care in terms of distance and travel time, in linkage with uptake of services and sometimes health or nutritional outcomes, have been widely documented in existing literature (Jones *et al.,* 1999; Soeung *et al.,* 2006). Studies in developing countries have shown that the absence of proper roads and lack of suitable communication networks particularly in the poor, remote and in adverse terrain constrain access to healthcare, food availability resulting in poor health outcomes of the population (Baker and Gesler, 2000; Rahman and Smith, 2000; Gupta *et al.*, 2003; Peters *et al.*, 2008; Mukherjee *et al.,* 2012). Hence the innovative measures for facilitating geographical accessibility are viewed having control over the increased level of market utilization and help in reducing vulnerabilities (Ayeni *et al.*, 1987; Rosero-Bixby, 2003; Victora *et al.*, 2003; Oppong and Hodgson, 2005).

The geographical challenges are part of the lives of the poor population in India who lives in remote hills, forest areas, islands and deserts, and subsist primarily on agriculture, fishing and collecting forest products. The highly complex topography coupled with poor road infrastructure, constrains the mobility of a large number of people (IIHMR, 2010; Dutta and Pant, 2003). The situation is more adverse in remote areas where people have to use multiple modes of transportation – boats, van rickshwas, and walk – to move from one place to another. As expected, the degree of difficulties rise manifold during monsoon season.

Climate Related Vulnerabilities

There exists a huge body of literature on chronic shocks like climate change and their impacts on human wellbeing. As it is evident, gradual change in climatic conditions is articulated through different forms like hurricanes, storms, floods, heat-waves and droughts, which are limited duration transient shocks (Naidoo, 2009). Extreme climatic events make poor inhabitants more vulnerable toother idiosyncratic or covariate shocks like health shocks as poor people are less resilient (Tanner and Mitchell, 2008). Earlier literatures related to well being of the people living in similar regions throughout the world view vulnerability of worsening of health and well being as a complex phenomenon. Accordingto them, vulnerability of a poor population increases as climatic shock brings health shocks, and the likelihood of further worsening of health status differs by inhabitants' resilience to chronic shocks, *i.e.*, coping capability they have and mechanism they adopt to rebuild affected economic and social conditions (Cutter *et al.,* 2003; Morrow, 1999). Threat of climatic shock as a result of climate change to undiversified livelihood and consequently on health through various routes is very common in areas like Latin American sub-continents as well as in some parts of south Asia like Vietnam, Bangladesh and India (Enarson, 2000; Omitsu and Yamano, 2006; Tanner and Mitchell, 2008; Tinh and Hang, 2003; Mukherjee *et al.,* 2012).

As found in vulnerable lives of the Amazon region—protein energy under-nutrition, intestinal parasitic infections, acute respiratory infection and iron deficiency are higher among poor and marginalized children whose families are victims of chronic climate shock (UNICEF, 2009). When climate events destroy intangible household resources the affected population becomes insecure with respect to food and shelter (Gregoryv *et al.*, 2005). Food insecurity ultimately causes under-nutrition through reduction in calorie intake. Moreover, after covariate-transient climatic shock, disease outbreaks cause lots of suffering alongwith food shortage (Shea, 2007). In climatic shock-prone areas, caregiver's knowledge about child care needs special attention as home management of child health shocks are differentfrom other areas (Skoufias *et al.*, 2011).

Health Related Vulnerabilities

In poverty stricken areas with insecure livelihood, girls experience early marriage and early child-bearing and without adequate nutrition and supplementation they remain or become undernourished which is indicated in earlier studies (Morales *et al.*, 2004). They give birth to low birth weight babies who become chronically undernourished in future (ibid.). Anecdotal evidences suggest that in the Sundarbans delta region in India, care givers are unable to provide adequate amount of diet and proper nature of diet at the appropriate time to their children due to their poor socioeconomic condition. Inaddition to this, sub-optimal healthcare service as well as lower acceptability of healthcare strengthens the under-nutrition morbidity vicious circle among children (Mukherjee *et al.*, 2012). As found in different shock-prone areas in the developing world, frequent occurrence of climatic events generate demand for efficient health and nutrition service availability with adequate supply of human resource where the system runs with sub-optimal capacity even in normal situations for providing effective service (WHO, 2005). Limited affordability, less social acceptability with improper knowledge and practice of childcare reduces the possibility of timely care for ailing children and make them vulnerable to under-nutrition (Andersen, 1995; Anderson and Davidson, 2001; Bradley *et al.*, 2002; Anderson 2008; Mukherjee 2014). Recurrent suffering from ailments due to less healthcare seeking increases the cost of care and sometimes hospitalization of acute cases increases the healthcare expenditure level of households in the absence of social protection (Dercon, 2005; Wagstaff and Doorslaer, 2001). Poor households having limited coping ability slips down into deeper poverty and becomes vulnerable to chronic poverty due to financial catastrophe (Doorslaer *et al.,* 2006).

In a nutshell, vulnerability is an output of exposure to hazard (shock) and the degree of resilience (Devereux *et al.,* 2006). Seasonality and crop failures, market volatility, disaster preceded morbidities, undiversified livelihood and limited ability to coping contributes to vulnerability. Limited financial and physical capital reduces the ability to cope with nature, human, epidemiology or insecurity related socks. Weak market chains, lower local import prices of goods produced or services offered by a particular area along with poor communication facility and costly transport aggravates local supply and demand shocks (Dorwardand Kydd, 2002). If shocks are multifaceted in nature and repeat from time to time, vulnerability becomes dynamic. As found in Malawi, at very initial phase, shocks and coping are mutually exclusive; over time recurring shocks weaken the resilience due to less effective coping or limited ability to assemble coping strategies (Sabates-Wheeler and Haddad, 2005). Therefore, weakening of resilience strengthens the vulnerabilities to multidimensional chronic poverty and poverty deepening. Combined policy measures including social insurance as well as safety net mechanisms can protect the vulnerable from destitution.

Currently, several development literatures deal with how climate change aggravates different natures of vulnerabilities and how to increase the effectiveness of investments in poverty eradication and sustainable development through reduction of such vulnerabilities. Frequent extreme weather event is one feature of climate change that destroys annual harvests, depletes fishing grounds, abolishes forests, make livelihoods insecure and households become highly sensitive and low resilient to such frequent shocks which results in deep rooted problem of highly prevalent chronic under-nutrition (The World Bank, 2009,

Mukherjee *et al.,* 2012). Economists, climate change specialists and development researchers suggest adaptation strengthening to climate change as the major instrument to build resilience. However, they also suggest that such low resilient regions or communities are in need of social protection or social risk management (Holzmann and Jorgensen, 1999; Mukherjee *et al.,* 2012).

As children are more vulnerable compared to other age groups, more focus on children living in such regions are required (Sanfilippo *et al.,* 2012). As per previous research, it can be done through evidence generation based on which investment on them can be made through social protection as return on such investment is quite high with respect to individual as well as society (Sanfilippo *et al.,* 2012; Asian Development Bank, 2001; Fajth, 2009; UNICEEF, 2009; Roetten and Sabates-Wheeler, 2011). Since, such protection, promotion and prevention will help to break intergenerational transfer of poverty and contribute to economic growth and reduce vulnerability (Sanfilippo *et al.,* 2012; Dercon, 2011).

2

Schools of Thought Regarding the Said Nexus

In health economics literature, many authoritative works consider whether there is any relation between ex ante, ex post economic status and under-nutrition (Devereux *et al.*, 2006; Dercon, 2005; Brennan *et al.*, 2004; Abeykoon, 1995; Bairagi, 1986; Briend *et al.*, 1988; Daulaire *et al.*, 1992; Elfindri, 1993; Esrey *et al.*, 1988; Lutter *et al.*, 1989; Mertens *et al.*, 1990; Pebley and Amin, 1991; Pelletier, 1994; Rahmathullah *et al.* 1990; Ruzicka and Kane, 1985; Schoenbaum *et al.*, 1995; Sommerfelt, 1991; Sommerfelt and Arnold, 1998; Sommerfelt and Stewart, 1994; Vella *et al.*, 1992a, Vijayaraghaven *et al.*, 1990; Visaria, 1987; West *et al.*, 1991; Zeger and Edelstein, 1989; Smith and Haddad, 1999; Ruel, 1999; Victora, 2008; Poel, 2008; Fotso, 2006; Hong and Mishra, 2006).

Authors analyzed the studies at population level, community level and individual level to assess the link between macro and micro level poverty and vulnerability with under-nutrition. In addition to this, vulnerability studies are disaggregated into nature of shocks, context of exposure and sectoral influence. I discuss all the studies under separate schools of thought or perspectives. I divide it into absolute income approach, absolute poverty or deprivation approach, relative poverty approach and ex ante poverty approach under one broader umbrella that follows materialistic approach.

ABSOLUTE INCOME APPROACH

Studies on inter and intra-country differential in under-nutrition depend on income growth of those countries (Smith and Haddad, 1999; Haddad *et al.,* 2003; Strauss and Thomas, 1998; Heltberg, 2009). They find under-nutrition prevalence is related to economic growth and growth elasticity of under-nutrition is as high as –0.50 both in macro and micro data. Therefore, their study proves the existence of inter-country inequality in under-nutrition depending upon the economic growth phenomenon. Heltberg (2009) shows the elasticity value much less, –0.20, since he uses stunting and Haddad (1999, 2003) uses underweight. Another important finding in literature is that economic growth impacts through the pathway of household standard of living *e.g.,* water and sanitation as well as demographic characteristics *e.g.,* fertility impact (Heady and Kohli, 2010). Another factor is dietary intake which influences growth-under-nutrition linkage. Literatures argue that diminishing returns to dietary intake on childhood under-nutrition is due to lack of dietary diversity (ibid.).

The reverse causality – impact of health on income – is also very important to understand the long run impact of population health on the economy. Health and nutrition of children influences their wage earning in future (Strauss and Thomas, 1998). Their works are on impact of health on income through the lens of labor economics. They analyze different experimental and quasi-experimental studies on impact of nutrition on income earning. One experimental study by Basta *et al.,* (1979) in Indonesia proves that in baseline anemic men were less productive than non-anemic men and at end-line, the intervention group becomes productive nearly equivalent to non-anemic workers. They also mention about one experimental study in Guatemala by Imminck and Viteri (1981a, 1981b) where productivity increased both in treatment and control group after intervention because researcher could not identify the experimental effect from village-time effect. Another study on Kenyan workers avoids this cavity where treatment effect shows a small positive impact of calorie supplementation

(Wolgemuth *et al.,* 1982). In Leibenstein's (1957) hypothesis, at low levels of calorie intake, association between better nutrition and higher labor productivity is visible. Higher labor productivity is expected to bring higher economic growth and therefore Strauss and Thomas (1998) argue that investment in health infrastructure and intervention that would help the economic growth through increase in labor productivity should be evaluated in this respect.

ABSOLUTE DEPRIVATION OR ABSOLUTE POVERTY APPROACH

As per deprivation approach, under-nutrition is a major public health concern in developing countries where it is a major cause and consequence of poverty (UNICEF, 1998; ACC/SCN, 1997). One study by Svedberg (2008) finds modest absolute poverty reduction is the cause of low rate of reduction in under-nutrition in a period of fifteen years in India. Though his aim was to see why economic growth failed to reduce under-nutrition average over this period, he finds poverty is the main factor along with mother's education and autonomy. His analysis is done at state level. The possibility of unobserved heterogeneity affecting the results is higher as he partially follows the basic framework on determinants of under-nutrition. Another point that needs attention is that he uses male female population ratio as a proxy for autonomy which is also a dubious point since quite a few other indicators like final say on money to be used, health care etc., are important dimensions to be considered under autonomy. Finally, he is not exploring the impact of state level idiosyncracies.

RELATIVE POVERTY APPROACH OR INCOME/ASSET INEQUALITY APPROACH

Different proximate and underlying determinants of nutritional status of the population in developing countries are responsible for huge gap in nutritional achievement between the rich and the poor (Wagstaff, 2002). According to Mosley and Chen (1984), Smith and Haddad (1999) and UNICEF framework (1990) there exist some proximate determinants *e.g.* dietary intake and health of the child and many underlying determinants of under-nutrition like socioeconomic status, healthcare provision, maternal education, maternal nutritional status, women's autonomy etc. which affect proximate determinants. Then further studies explore there are few basic factors, which influence those underlying factors from macro level.

Immediate or proximate determinants of childhood under-nutrition are poor dietary intake of the child and his poor health which are individual level factors. Timely initiation of complementary feeding and exclusive breastfeeding are significantly worse across developing countries, and especially among the poor households within those countries (Wagstaff *et al.,* 2003).

Underlying determinants are household and community level factors. Child feeding practice, preventive care, care for small children and care during childbirth, environment where the child lives (like place of defecation, source of drinking water, living in kutcha house, having no separate kitchen, using biomass fuel for cooking and heating), mother's knowledge, household's food security, access to health facility are underlying determinants which indirectly influence childhood nutritional status *via* their impact on proximate determinants (Svedberg, 2000; Onis *et al.,* 2000; Chakrabarty, 2004; Navaneetham and Jose, 2005; Linnermayr *et al.,* 2008; Svedberg, 2008; Aturupane *et al.,* 2008; Pongou *et al.,* 2006; Taguri *et al.,* 2008; Setboonsarng, 2005; IIPS, 2007; Mishra and Ratherford, 2000). All these correlates show unequal distribution among the poor and the rich (ibid.).

The basic determinant, which affects all the underlying determinants, is poverty at macro level (Smith and Haddad, 1999) *i.e.,* at national or state level if considered in DH sense. From DH perspective it is headcount ratio but in relative poverty sense it is individual, community or population level rich-poor gap whether measured in income/consumption metrics or asset possession.

Schools of Thought Regarding the Said Nexus

Different earlier works explore the link between economic status and under-nutrition (Deolalikar, 2004; Svedberg, 2000; Navaneetham and Jose, 2005; Hong and Mishra, 2006; Svedberg, 2008). These studies argue that there exists a two-way causality between economic status and under-nutrition as poor people are more undernourished and under-nutrition reduces production of human capital and in the long run reduces work capacity and earning (Dasgupta and Roy, 1986).

In Asian countries like Bangladesh, India, range of Latin American and sub-Saharan African countries living standard and children's nutritional status are interrelated (Poel *et al.,* 2008; Zere and McIntyre, 2003; Fotso, 2006; Hong and Mishra, 2006; Smith and Haddad, 1999; Pongou *et al.,* 2006; Larrea and Freire, 2002; Taguri *et al.,* 2008; Giashuddin *et al.,* 2005). But in countries like Mexico, Ecuador, Cambodia any relation between economic status and under-nutrition is absent (Hong *et al.,* 2006). Economic status, healthcare and regional characteristics are a few determinants of under-nutrition in Ghana (Poel *et al.,* 2007). In some developing countries, income growth improves nutrition outcomes but the trickle-down effect is slow, long and indirect (Shekar and Lee, 2006).

Economic status is one correlate which influences the decision making of the household related to children's share of food in the family as well as health seeking at household level (Tipping and Segall, 1996; Linnermayr *et al.,* 2008). One study finding shows that a child from the richest quintile is twice as likely to be taken to a suitable provider compared to a poor child when suffering from diarrhoea or pneumonia (Gwatkin *et al.,* 2000). Such adherences are strongly associated with socioeconomic status of the households found in rural Sudan also (Wagstaff *et al.,* 2003). Another study on Tanzania shows that poorer children are significantly less likely to receive antibiotics when they suffer from pneumonia (Schellenberg *et al.,* 2003).

Therefore, economic status *via* household's behavior influences intra-household food allocation, preventive and curative care seeking which influences child's health and nutritional status. These literatures also measure the impact of economic status and different economists recommend several policy directions to reduce the impacts and protect children from those impacts.

A World Bank study argues that poverty reduction strategy process will be strengthened if emphasis is laid on nutrition (Shekar and Lee, 2006). Poverty reduction will then be accelerated as improved nutrition will accelerate future human capital development (Shekar and Lee, 2006). Since the poor are more undernourished, therefore if nutritional interventions target those groups then it will reduce the prevalence of undernourishment and will break the vicious circle of under-nutrition and poverty (Shekar and Lee, 2006). Thus poverty reduction along with nutritional interventions will improve the health and well-being of the poor (Setboonsarng, 2005; Shekar and Lee, 2006).

Despite such thinking of and actions by donor organizations, it is prominent that the childhood under-nutrition is still a considerable problem in Asian countries. Notwithstanding lower incidence of poverty, South Asia shows higher prevalence of undernourished children in the world (Navaneetham and Jose, 2005). In South Asia, 40 percent population is under lower poverty line as defined by the World Bank compared to 46.3 percent in Sub Saharan Africa whereas, incidence of under-nutrition is higher in South Asia compared to Sub Saharan Africa (Moderate to severe stunting in South Asia is 44.8 percent compared to 32.8 percent in Sub Saharan Africa) (Navaneetham and Jose, 2005; Svedberg, 2000). One study projects that India will take until 2023 to achieve the MDGs under the best of circumstances (Shekar and Lee, 2006). In India currently 26 percent population is below poverty line but 38 percent child population is undernourished (NHDR, 2001; IIPS, 2007). Despite a number of poverty eradication programmes and nutritional interventions in India under-nutrition rate is so high (Gragnolati *et al.,* 2005).

Not only the economic status, poverty syndrome factors at individual, household and community level play important role in determining child's nutritional status (Navaneetham and Jose, 2005). As for example, child nutrition is influenced by urbanization (Navaneetham and Jose, 2005; Fotso, 2006). Demographic factor related to household like household size is another determinant of under-nutrition (Navaneetham and Jose, 2005; Taguri *et al.,* 2008; Mamobolo *et al.,* 2005).

Frequency of childhood illness also depends on whether the feeding practice is not proper (Wagstaff *et al.,* 2003). From the very first hour of birth to five months of age exclusive breastfeeding protects the child on or after suffering from infectious diseases and under-nutrition (WHO, 2001). From six months onwards only breast milk is not able to provide sufficient nutrition and energy to combat with diseases but children need frequent, consistent complementary feeding following proper feeding approach along with breastfeeding (Wagstaff, 2003). Improper start of complementary feeding has different negative consequences (ibid.). Per capita food availability, food security in the household is another underlying determinant affecting the dietary intake of children in the household (Smith and Haddad, 1999; Yambi and Kavishe, 1999; Garcia, 1994; Onis *et al.,* 2000). In India, eminent economists feel that properly working Public Distribution System (PDS) is needed to bring food security (Swaminathan, 2001). Given the equitable intra-household food allocation, poorer households will benefit from efficient food distribution through PDS than food production due to rising role of market in agriculture (ibid.). A significant shock to the children at their age of less than three has discernible impacts ten years later in terms of height achievement. This perpetuates inequality in future (Zere and McIntyre, 2003).

Access to public goods and services *e.g.,* drinking water, toilet and sanitation facility determines household's environment which have influence on child's nutritional status in a family which is one community and household level determinant (Svedberg, 2000; Monteiro *et al.,* 2009; Onis *et al.,* 2000; Linnermayr *et al.,* 2008; Taguri *et al.,* 2008; Navaneetham and Jose, 2005; Kavishe and Yambi, 1999; Hong and Mishra, 2006). Place of defecation, hand washing after defecation or before cooking, safe drinking water influence the occurrence of diarrhoea and other infectious diseases (Wagstaff, 2003). Water and sanitation act as underlying determinants because they have an impact on proximate determinants like feeding of the child which is affected by the quality of drinking water and sanitation (Wagstaff, 2003, Linnemayr *et al.*, 2008). Indoor Air Pollution due to use of coal or biomass fuels (wood, animal dung etc.) for cooking or heating without proper ventilation increases the risk of pneumonia among children and birth of low birth weight babies (Wagstaff, 2003).

Preventive activities like antenatal visits, health worker's advice about mother and child's nutrition are community level characteristics that improve mother's nutritional status, reduce the probability of low birth weight babies and promote proper feeding practice of mother and children (Wagstaff, 2003). Studies show that less healthcare uptake as indicated by incomplete immunization worsens impacts of under-nutrition, and also found to be the significant risk factor for stunting (Taguri *et al.*, 2008).

Care during illness is a household level underlying determinant (Haddad *et al.*, 1995; Martorell *et al.*, 1984). Poor or delayed care seeking is found as the cause of 70 percent of child deaths (Wagstaff, 2003). Knowledge about the symptoms and danger signs of severe illness influences the decision of taking to a right provider (ibid.).

Financial barrier of the poor is one household level obstacle, which not only means less resource to combat health shock but also the economic impact of seeking treatment (Russell, 2004). Poor people's monthly consumption is highly responsive to health seeking. Single hospital utilization in Vietnam in 1998 cost 22 percent of annual non-food consumption expenditure for the poorest quintile (Wagstaff and Doorslaer, 2003). Poorest people in India curtail 60 percent of food consumption when they utilize hospital care (Kanjilal *et al.*, 2007).

Healthcare provision at community level means a lot of issues - geographical accessibility, availability of human resources, organizational and technical quality, relevance and timeliness of services. Distance and time to reach health facility has significant impact on service use and health status outcome and poor people usually have to travel more to get a healthcare service and they also face difficulty in transportation (Wagstaff, 2003). Utilization of services is higher in households where healthcare services are well-equipped with machinery, drug stock and properly staffed and the study also finds that facilities serving the poor are not well staffed nor well stocked (Wagstaff, 2003). The poor usually become a victim of improper organizational quality while they go to public facilities and suffer from long waiting or rude behavior (Wagstaff, 2003). Poor people visit hospitals, which are of inferior organizational quality, and quality of case management of childhood illness is frequently very low (WHO, 1998).

Child's nutritional intake, intra household food allocation, health care seeking of children depend upon one crucial household level factor - mother's education which influences her knowledge, awareness, and also decision-making power (Svedberg, 2000; Onis *et al.,* 2000; Chakrabarty, 2004; Navaneetham and Jose, 2005; Linnermayr *et al.* 2008; Svedberg, 2008; Aturupane *et al.,* 2008; Pongou *et al.,* 2006; Taguri *et al.,* 2008). Child's under-nutrition decreases with increase in mother's education, as educated mothers are more likely to follow better feeding practice, more likely to avail preventive and curative healthcare services and do proper childcare (Wagstaff, 2003; Linnermayr *et al.,* 2008). Across country and within country inequality in maternal education is substantial particularly in South Asia and western and central Africa. Parental poverty and low educational attainment are adversely associated with the survival of children as found in few other studies on under-nutrition (Montgomery and Hewett, 2005; Victora *et al.,* 2003).

Maternal nutritional status is significant household level influencing factor for child's growth retardation as many studies reflect (Chakrabarty, 2004; Morales *et al.,* 2004; Mani, 2007; Black *et al.,* 2008). Women who were undernourished as children are likely to give birth to low birth weight babies (Setboonsarng, 2005;

Navaneetham and Jose, 2005). South Asia is the worst in this respect (Poel *et al.,* 2008). Low birth weight is one of the main causes of higher prevalence of under-nutrition as girls and women are less well cared (1/3 of Indian babies, ½ of Bangladeshi babies are born low birth weight) (Navaneetham and Jose, 2005). It reflects gender dimension also. Again, low birth weight not only predicts poorer health in early childhood but also predicts suffering from chronic degenerative diseases (especially the risk of high glucose concentration, high blood pressure, high lipid profiles, and mental illness) in adulthood (Navaneetham and Jose, 2005, Victora *et al.,* 2008). Negative attitude of families towards mother's autonomy largely affects maternal health outcomes in the poor community, and in this manner affects time and energy that mothers devote for childcare and health seeking (Svedberg, 2008).

As I see, different studies try to understand whether the influencing factors are clustered in different levels like state, community, household, and individual. Alderman (2006) considers a few underlying influencing factors from individual level (child), mother, household and community level (presence of NGO and public health facility but not the utilization of those facilities due to data limitation) to understand the same.

One study by Linnemayr, Alderman and Ka (2008) on 12 developing countries to measure how far income change can reduce under-nutrition shows that countries with higher per capita income have less under-nutrition. They estimate the short term, medium term and long term impact of income change on the prevalence of under-nutrition and find that estimates of income effects are more sensitive to treatment of unobserved community factors compared to controls for household's access to public good.

Alderman (2006) considers the interaction between different level factors – maternal characteristics (early childbearing and maternal education) and presence of NGO in Senegal in influencing child's nutritional outcome - to explore the causality that may be suppressed by averaging of the data (total effect may not represent the group specific effects). He finds that young mothers are most likely to get benefited from services of NGOs and health facilities compared to older mothers. Different economists consider interaction between proximate and underlying determinants or two underlying determinants to find the disaggregated effects on child's anthropometric status. Caldwell's (1979) study shows a complementary relation between two underlying determinants - mother's education and health services. Rosenzweig and Schultz (1982) argue that availability of health facility reduces the inequality in health seeking behavior due to education implying substitutability between the presence of health facility and impact of mother's education on utilization of medical care. Alderman's (2006) Senegal study also finds substitutability among presence of health service post and mother's level of education. Barrera (1990) finds substitutability between mother's education and water connection and community cleanliness but a complementarity between maternal education and toilet connection in Philippines.

Under relative poverty approach a number of studies address the spatial (rural urban) inequalities in under-nutrition prevalence to find inequality at community level and they use mainly logistic regression techniques to find the correlates of inequality as well as determinants of under-nutrition at urban and rural level.

On an average, child health conditions are better in urban areas than in rural counterparts in developing countries (Poel *et al.,* 2007; Ruel *et al.,* 1998; Menon *et al.,* 2000; Fotso and Kuate-Defo, 2006). Improvement of understanding about the nature and the causes of rural urban disparities is essential to assess the impact of rapid urbanization taking place in the developing world in order to target resources appropriately to raise population health (Poel *et al.,* 2007). Different studies argue that, the locus of poverty and under-nutrition is shifting from rural area to urban area (Ruel and Garrett, 1999; Garrett, 2000). Poel (2007) finds that the urban poor have higher level of stunting than the rural poor in some developing countries. In some of the Sub-Saharan African countries, rural-urban differential in under-nutrition is narrowing due to increase in urban percentage and widening in some because of sharp decline in urban under-nutrition (Fotso, 2006). A study on different cities of Africa, Asia and Latin America finds spatial clustering of childhood under-nutrition and its covariates (Morris, 2000). In a study of nutritional status of children under the age of five in Mozambique, Garrett (1999) and Ruel (1999) show that it is the levels of critical influencing factors and not their nature that are responsible for rural-urban differential in under-nutrition and food insecurity. Another study also concludes the same (Smith *et al.,* 2004).

The aforementioned studies investigated different correlates of rural-urban differential in under-nutrition. Among those correlates, household wealth is one strong determinant of rural-urban disparity (Poel *et al.,* 2007). Greater dependence on cash income, employment in informal sector, and greater exposure to environmental contamination are major causes in addition to the previous one (Ruel *et al.,* 1999). Most common causes of under-nutrition are poor feeding practice, less utilization of nutrients due to infections and parasites, inadequate food and health security, poor environmental conditions, and lack of proper child care practice (Ghosh and Shah, 2004). In one study, Ruel (2000) finds that in Latin America, rural children are worse off in terms of growth and dietary diversity than their urban counterpart. He also shows that exclusive breastfeeding up to five months and complementary feeding from 6 months are key concerns of urban area. Though breastfeeding rates are lower in urban areas, dietary patterns are better as urban mothers are more likely to start complementary feeding in timely fashion (Ruel and Menon, 2002). In Sub-Saharan Africa and South Asia, under-nutrition largely is a material dimension of poverty including water and sanitation, access to food and healthcare along with the crucial factor income, mother's education and maternal nutritional status in alleviating child under-nutrition which has strong and significant community level variance (Fotso and Firestone, 2008; Fotso, 2006; Harttgen and Misselhorn, 2006). In Poel's (2007) study, controlling for socio-demographic characteristics reduces rural-urban risk ratio by 22 percent implying that demographic characteristics also have significant influence on the economic gradient of rural-urban differential in under-nutrition (Poel *et al.,* 2007). In Sub-Saharan Africa, after controlling for economic status, the rural-urban gap disappears implying that focus is needed for urban poor children (Fotso, 2006). Identification of factors affecting the health of urban poor and programs that target them are very urgent in phase of urbanization (Poel *et al.,* 2007; Ruel *et al.,* 1999). Besides, Efforts to alleviate the most critical socioeconomic constraints specific to the different environment should continue to be prioritized (Smith *et al.,* 2005).

There is considerable intra-urban heterogeneity in economic condition and under-nutrition (Ruel *et al.,* 1998). The nutritional status of slum children is worst among all urban dwellers and is even poorer than the rural average (Ghosh and Shah, 2004; Magadi, 2004). When such degree of under-nutrition among urban poor combines with morbidity then it causes complexities in designing, targeting and implementing urban programmes (Ruel and Garrett, 2004). Using 85 DHS urban samples Montgomery and Hewett (2005) show that household and neighbourhood (whether household is living in an area where concentration of poverty/affluence is present) living standard has significant influence on children's height for age.

Lack of health and public services, decreased breastfeeding due to maternal employment, maternal malnutrition and poor health leading to reduced capacity of mothers to perform care-giving activities are the main causes of long persistent higher intra-urban differential in under-nutrition which sometimes seems higher than rural-urban differential (Timaeus and Lush, 1995; Ruel *et al.,* 1998; Ruel *et al.,* 1999). These factors are interrelated in their effects and their relative importance as well as size of intra-urban differential varies greatly between countries (Timaeus and Lush, 1995). Magadi (2004) shows that lower educational achievements are consistently associated with poor health achievements of urban poor in Kenya. A study in urban slum in

India shows that prolonged breastfeeding, late introduction of complementary feeding are responsible for poor nutritional status of children (Kapur *et al.,* 2005). In an 11 country study to see whether intra-urban differential in child stunting is higher than intra-rural differential, authors find that stunting is lower in urban area than rural area but inequality in nutritional status is higher in urban area (Menon *et al.,* 2000). In developing countries, poor urban households are much less likely than other urban households to enjoy access to public services (Hewett and Montgomery, 2001). Urban slum children in Kenya are less likely to be fully immunized and more likely to suffer from fever and diarrhoea (Magadi, 2004).

Failure to appropriately target the growing subgroup of urban poor and failure to improve their living conditions and health status may result in lack of improvement in national indicators of health (Fotso *et al.,* 2007). Applying data from Guatemalan Survey of Family Health, Heuveline and Goldman (2000) show that modern medical care plays a major role in treatment of undernourished sick children in rural Guatemala. Effective governance can bring integrated public health and nutrition efforts with other Government agencies to improve health by spatial distribution in low and middle income countries (Montgomery, 2009). Since urban health system is very complex with presence of private for-profit and non-profit care, Montgomery (2009) suggests effective partnership with them. Hewett and Montgomery (2001) suggest that continuous public sector investment in service delivery will help to eradicate less health service uptake among urban poor.

EX ANTE POVERTY APPROACH OR VULNERABILITY AND UNDER-NUTRITION

Vulnerability to poverty and under-nutrition is previously analyzed from consumption and investment poverty perspective. Studies show that the association between vulnerability to consumption poverty concept and under-nutrition gets affected byperception and beliefs of caregivers in underdeveloped economies. Therefore, though likelihood of future status fall describes the inequality in nutritional status, this factor is not sufficient to explain the vulnerability to become under-nourished. Service delivery effectiveness and availability of good quality care is major important factor to reduce vulnerability to be under-nourished as people face out of pocket expenses more relying on unqualified practitioners. According to the investment poverty perspective, likelihood of stunting is higher among more contextually vulnerable subgroup.

Regarding vulnerability to consumption poverty, it is usually visible in other developing countries that vulnerable less-poor families are more prone to transient bouts of poverty after any shock (Zaman, 1998; Zaman, 2000). In a few pockets of India, when poorer families face climatic shock induced health shocks like diarrhea among their children, they first visit nearby unqualified providers due to local connections, trust and availability of treatment either in credit or in package system as found in earlier studies (IIHMR, 2010). But as it is evident in one study, some of them experience worsening of child's health or recurrence of the disease and therefore search for costlier private provider because service of Government facility is sub-optimal in quantity. The study also shows that the cost they incur for treatment doubles and they cope with such situation through consumption sacrifice as safety nets are almost unavailable. Such a situation makes them vulnerable to future poverty as also evident in previous studies in rural Ethiopia or Vietnam (Calvo and Dercon, 2005; Wagstaff and Doorslaer, 2000).

On the other hand, households who face asset loss due to climatic shock and low resilient due to living under extreme poverty, they even cannot go for any treatment options after such health shocks but rely on home remedies to cure the child. Though due to good social cohesion, traditional knowledge and beliefs for treatment are shared among each other but this is not sufficient to break the under-nutrition morbidity vicious circle, especially when the under-nutrition is chronic in nature as visible in supporting qualitative study. Supporting this argument, as found in an in-depth anthropological study on variation in the household management of child diarrhea in 3 villages in rural North India; qualitative and quantitative results showed both positive and negative diarrhea management behaviors where the study used to collect data on a series of variables, including maternal knowledge, beliefs, and practices during diarrhea, feeding and fluid intake during diarrhea, treatment choices, and knowledge and use of oral rehydration therapy (Bentley, 1988).

Hence vulnerability due to health shocks remains crucial for developing nations like India in the absence of safety net measures that might have protected the households from being vulnerable to such health shocks; more specifically for the ones those share weak endowments. Side by side, Vulnerability to worse health and nutritional status preceded by asset loss due to big covariate shock *e.g.*, climatic shock or consumption sacrifice due to idiosyncratic health shock or this idiosyncratic consumption shock if is preceded by that large investment shock make households vulnerable to poverty – transient or chronic- as well as such economic vulnerabilities make the child population vulnerable to chronic under-nutrition. Therefore as per vulnerability sub-groups, specific policy focuses are required to shatter the poverty-vulnerability – chronic under-nutrition-morbidity vicious circle.

The Indian Context

Despite recent achievement in economic progress in India (World Bank, 2003), the fruit of development fails to secure a better nutritional status of children in the country (Rajaram *et al.*, 2007; Shiva Kumar, 2007; Pathak and Singh, 2009; Svedberg, 2006). India presents a typical scenario of South-Asia, fitting the adage of 'Asian Enigma' (Ramalingaswami *et al.*, 1996); where progress in childhood under-nutrition seems to have sunk into an apparent under-nutrition trap, lagging far behind other Asian countries characterized by similar levels of economic development (Gragnolati *et al.*, 2005; UNICEF, 1990; Svedberg, 2007; Claeson *et al.*, 2000).

In the light of above analysis of literatures, I shall look into the Indian scenario in an in-depth manner. Exhibiting a sluggish declining trend over the past decade and a half, the recent estimate from the National Family Health Survey -3 (NFHS-3) - the unique source for tracking the status of child under-nutrition in India (Mishra and Rutherford, 2000) - indicates that about 38 percent are moderately to severely stunted (short for age) (IIPS, 2007). The decline in prevalence however becomes unimpressive with the average levels marked by wide inequality in childhood under-nutrition across the states and various socioeconomic groups (Rajaram *et al.*, 2007; Shiva Kumar, 2007; Bawdekar and Ladusingh, 2008). Growing evidence suggests (Pathak and Singh, 2009) that in India the gap in prevalence of under-nutrition among rich and poor children is increasing over the years with wide regional differentials. From this specific context, my work is an attempt to study the pattern of the nutritional status of Indian children in last few decades as well as the pattern in the local context incorporating uncertainty.

Socioeconomic differences in morbidity and mortality rates across the world have received its due attention in recent years (Wagstaff, 2000a; Brockerhoff and Hewett, 2000; Gilson and McIntyre, 2001). Such differentials in health status in-fact are pervasive across nations' cross-cutting stages of development as mentioned above (Mohanty and Pathak, 2009; Poel *et al.*, 2008; Houweling *et al.*, 2007; Lawn *et al.*, 2006; Carr, 2004; Gwatkin *et al.*, 2004; Oomann *et al.*, 2003; Zere and McIntyre, 2003; Wagstaff, 2002; Wagstaff, 2000b; Gwatkin *et al.*, 2007; Smith and Haddad, 1999). Studies identify that poverty is the chief determinant of under-nutrition in developing countries that perpetuates into intergenerational under-nutrition and prevents social improvement and equity (Larrea and Kawachi, 2005; Hong *et al.*, 2006). Literature also considers nutritional status of under-five children in particular as one of the most important indicators of a household's living standard and also an important determinant of child survival (Thomas *et al.*, 1990). The deterministic studies in India while exploring the impact of covariates on degree of childhood under-nutrition come up with an important nexus shared between household socioeconomic status and under-nutrition (ICMR, 1972; Rao and Rao, 1994; Rajaram *et al.*, 2003; Rao *et al.*, 2004; Bamji, 2003; Bharati, 2008; Pal, 1999; Zere and McIntyre, 2003; Rajaram *et al.*, 2007; Arnold *et al.*, 2004; Radhakrishna and Ravi, 2004). The two-way causality of poverty and under-nutrition seems to pose a very significant pretext for under-nutrition in India like other developing nations, where poverty and economic insecurity due to constrained access to economic resources permeate undernourishment among the children (Behrman and Deolalikar, 1988; World Development Report, 1993; Strauss and Thomas, 1998; World Health Report 1999; Ruger and Kim, 2006, Gragnolati *et. al.*, 2005). Thus, economic deprivation and inequality constitute the focal point of discussion while studying under-nutrition and deserve suitable analytical treatment to examine their interplay with other dimensions of under-nutrition and to prioritize appropriate programme intervention. This kind of nexus in a world of uncertainty needs further attention and less explored till now in the context of developing world. The present work tries to fill up the existing gap with respect to India and one local context.

3

Blend of Health Capital and Behavioural Models: The Conceptual Framework

In poverty stricken area, the nutrition capital production of population subgroup is different from general nutrition capital production model. The theoretical model in this chapter is based on Grossman's (1972) demand for health concept. Economists derive nutrition demand function from household's utility function. Current theoretical model is the contextualized version of Smith and Haddad (2000). The household behaves as if maximizing a welfare function, *W*, made up of the utility functions of its members (*Ui*), indexed *i*= 1, ..., *n*. The household members include a care giver who is assumed to be the mother (indexed *i*= *M*), *D* other adults (indexed *i*= 1, ...,*D*), and *J* children (indexed *i*= 1, ..., *J*).

The welfare function takes the form:

$$W\,(U_M, U^1{}_{ad}, \ldots\ldots, U^D{}_{ad}, U^1{}_{ch}, \ldots, U^J{}_{ch} \beta \text{ and } \beta = (\beta M, \beta^1{}_{ad}, \ldots, \beta^D{}_{ad}) \qquad (1)$$

where the βs represent each adult household member's "status." Such status affects the relative weight placed on members' preferences in overall household decision-making, or their decision-making power.

The utility functions take the form:

$$U^i = U(N, F, X_0, T_L)\ i=1,\ldots\ldots,n \qquad (2)$$
$$i=1+D+J$$

where N, F, Xo and T_L are $1 X N$ vectors of the nutritional status, food and non-food consumption, and leisure time of each household member.

Nutritional status is viewed as a household provisioning process with inputs of food, non-food commodities and services, and care. The nutrition provisioning function for child i is as follows:

$$N^i_{ch} = N(F^i, C^i, X^i_N, ?_{HENV} X^i_{FOOD}, X^i_{MEDU}, X^i_{HEXP} F^i)\ i=1,\ldots\ldots.J \qquad (3)$$

Where F^i is the food received by the ith child and C^i is the care received by the ith child, X^i_N represents non-food commodities and services purchased for care giving purposes, such as health services. In respect of blending this concept with Andersen's model, I also incorporate the health seeking behaviour related factors in this group *e.g.* personal health choices, choice of providers, perceived quality of care, perceived health and nutritional status of children and related perceived necessities of accessing care.

The variable F^i_{HENV} represents the health environment, that is, the availability of safe water, sanitation, in the household's community which is supposed to influence other different predisposing and enabling factors.

The variable $?_{FOOD}$ represents the availability of food in the community. Finally, the variable $?_{MEDU}$ represents the mother's educational status which influences her knowledge, attitudes, beliefs and practice regarding child care which is the household capital that falls under the subgroup of predisposing factors as per Andersen's model. The child's care, C^i, is itself treated as a child-specific, household- provisioned service depends on mother's decision-making process in care giving which is assumed to be governed by her education level (assumed to be contemporaneously exogenous). This factor is an enabling factor (ibid.). The term $?^i$

indicates the physiological endowment of the child (his or her innate healthiness), cultural factors affecting caring practices; the mother's own nutritional status embodying the status of her physical and mental health, Household members' income constraint is reflected in their economic status. This set of factors is an endowment of predisposing and enabling factors and all these different sets influence the "need" of health and nutrition capital production *i.e.* generation of individual to aggregate effective demand. Such demand for nutrition and health supposed to influence household's utility maximization and finally maximization of individual and collective welfare subject to household and community level utility maximization would suppose to take place.

In a world with uncertainty, several covariate and idiosyncratic shocks influence everyday human life. As for an example, frequent extreme climatic events distort the physical environment through contamination of drinking water, increase in risk of infection through improper sanitation; disrupting household and community assets through devastations; increasing the risk of morbidity and side by side water logging and other destructions upset the physical accessibility. In addition to all these, such kind of shocks make livelihoods insecure, discontinuity in school attendance, interruption in everyday childcare due to unavailability of resources and many more. Then how the above mentioned theoretical model will behave is the point of analysis in this book. Therefore the new sustainable model will be developed considering the risks and uncertainties so that the welfare of vulnerable communities can be maximized.

THE ANALYTICAL FRAMEWORK

The analytical framework depicts the conceptual one in a contextual format where it tries to correlate how different barriers to adaptation and mitigation retards long term nutritional achievement of children within the vulnerable communities. Health

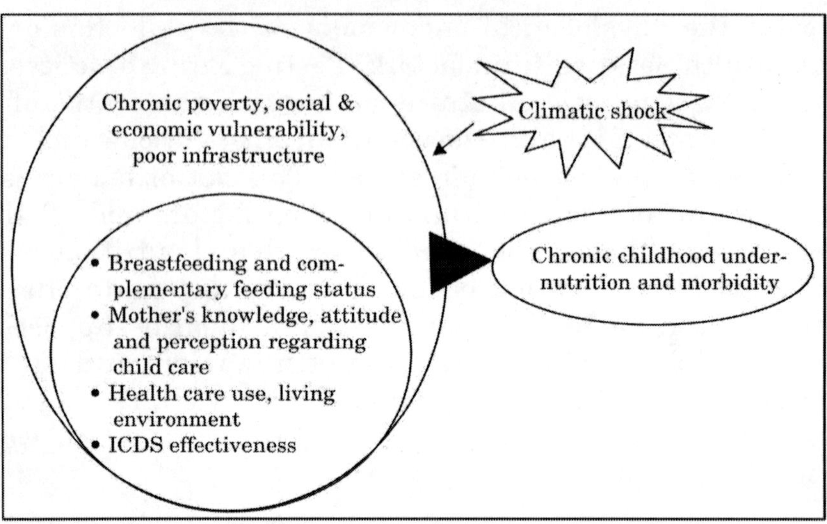

Source: Partially adopted from Haddad, 1999.

and socioeconomic as well as environmental adaptation *i.e.*, adapting to climate induced health and other idiosyncratic shock through overcoming the barriers help population to maintain a health status quo (Moser and Ekstrom, 2010). Based on traditional framework of under-nutrition determinants I can frame the situation according to our context. Childhood chronic under-nutrition is hypothesized to be influenced by some proximate and underlying factors as well as some distal factors. Here I take child's dietary intake (breastfeeding and complementary feeding practice) as proximate factors. Mother's knowledge attitude about childcare and perception regarding child's nutritional status, mother and child's healthcare use, living environment and in the supply side the ICDS effectiveness is taken as the underlying factors. Along with all this, the basic determinants in the vulnerable areas are chronic poverty, livelihood insecurity, socioeconomic vulnerabilities and poor infrastructure which are overarching all the determinants. And the major contextual influencing factor may be frequent climatic shocks due to climate change which affects all the above mentioned factors. I will explore how the complex pathway of interaction between the factors retards adaptation.

4

Pattern of Inequity from Demand – Supply Perspective: Influence of Context in India

Following previous analysis of developing countries as well as Indian context, in this chapter I am bringing an evidence based presentation of current Indian scenario comparing last one and half decades. I will explore;

1. Whether socioeconomic gradient of under-nutrition in India became stronger in last one and half decades,
2. Factors contributing to the inequity in nutritional status and the degree of contribution
3. Whether the amount of contributions are changing over the time and whether varies across states.

DATA AND METHODS

My work focuses on the objectives using Demographic and Health Survey data on India for three rounds. NFHS I, NFHS II, and NFHS III are designed to provide estimates of important maternal and child health indicators including nutritional status for young children (under three years are included for data comparability), following standard anthropometric components. The surveys are conducted following stratified sampling technique, details on the sampling procedure can be found at IIPS, 1994, 2000, 2007. Of the total children for whom NFHS I, NFHS II and NFHS III has similar information, a subset of 48,640 children are considered; those who are under the age of three and whose height-for-age z-score (HAZ) is available within the range of -6 to +6 standard deviation from the WHO-NCHS reference population for fifteen major states. I analysc in two phases – first, I see the socioeconomic gradient in India in three time points and then for four state groups where the grouping is based on the result of one previous work by Kanjilal *et al.* (2010). In this work fifteen major states are clubbed in four groups based on the NSDP, state prevalence of chronic under-nutrition (stunting) and state level concentration index values indicating inequity in nutritional status in those states for the year 2005-06. According to such categorization, four groups are: 1) High Prevalent High Inequity (HPHI) state: Orissa, 2) High Prevalent Moderate Inequity (HPMI) state: Andhra Pradesh, Tamil Nadu, Karnataka, Gujarat, 3) High Prevalent Low Inequity (HPLI) state: Rajasthan, Uttar Pradesh, Madhya Pradesh, Bihar, Assam, and 4) Moderate Prevalent High Inequity (MPHI) state: Haryana, Punjab, West Bengal, Maharashtra, Kerala.

I use three major methods for studying the objectives. The objective of calculating inequity in nutritional status is catered through the measurement of concentration index. To do the cluster wise analysis for exploring the factors influencing stunting and socioeconomic gradient in three time points I use multilevel modeling technique. And next to find the magnitude of contribution of different factors in inequity in nutritional status I use the technique of concentration index decomposition following O'Donnell *et al.* (2008).

CONCENTRATION INDEX

The widely used standard tool that examines the magnitude of economic inequality in any health outcome, *i.e.,* Concentration Index (CI) (O'Donnell *et al.,* 2008) is employed to study the extent of inequity in chronic child under-nutrition across the states of India.

The tool has been universally used by the economists to measure the degree of inequality in various health system indicators, such as health outcome, health care utilization and financing (O'Donnell *et al.*, 2008).

The value of CI ranges between -1 to +1, hence, if there is no economic differential the value is zero. A negative value implies that the relevant health variable is concentrated among the poor or disadvantaged people while the opposite is true for its positive values, when poorest are assigned the lowest value of the wealth index. A zero CI implies a state of horizontal equity which is defined as equal treatment for equal needs (O'Donnell *et al.*, 2008). CI values calculated for stunting help us find the possible concentration among rich and poor children below three years of age during NFHS I, II and III.

MULTI-LEVEL REGRESSION

Due to the stratified nature of data in NFHS (IIPS & ORC Macro 2007) the children are naturally nested into mothers, mothers are nested into households, and households are into states. Hence keeping in view this hierarchically clustered nature, the work uses multi-level regression model to estimate parameter for nutritional status among children to avoid the likely under-estimation of parameters from a single level model (Griffith *et al.*, 2002). Since siblings are expected to share certain common characteristics of the mother (mother's education), household (religion, caste) and community (availability of health facilities and outcomes); I can reasonably claim that unobserved heterogeneity in the outcome variable is also correlated at the cluster levels (Rice and Jones, 1997; Bingenheimer and Raudenbush, 2004; Marini and Gragnolati, 2006). This amounts to an estimation problem employing conventional OLS estimators, which gives efficient estimates only when the community (village/town) level covariates and the household level covariates are uncorrelated with the individual and maternal covariates.

Researchers adopt fixed effects models to estimate nutrition models and control for unobservable variables at the cluster level, which leads to the difficulty that if the fixed effect is differenced away, then the effect of those variables that do not vary within a cluster will be lost in the estimation process (Marini and Gragnolati, 2006). Iinvestigate whether the contextual factors influence the impact of household standard of living on child under-nutrition through random effect of household and community to see whether household and community level variation in prevalence of stunting is increasing adopting multilevel models.

We test one type of multilevel models; the variance components (random intercept) models. I use STATA routines for hierarchical linear models using maximum likelihood estimators for linear mixed models (Skrondal and Hesketh, 2007). The variance-components model correct for the problem of correlated observations in a cluster, by introducing a random effect at each cluster. In other words, subjects within the same cluster are allowed to have a shared random intercept. I consider two clusters, namely, community and household, since in most of the cases NFHS provides information on children of one mother chosen from a particular household. Thus, I have,

$$z_{jk} = \beta 2\ x_{jk} + \delta_j + €_{jk}$$

where z_{jk} is the HAZ score for the child(ren) from the kth household in the jth PSU. β is a vector of regression coefficients corresponding to the effects of fixed covariates x_{jk}, which are the observed characteristics of the child, the mother, the household and the community. Where, j' is a random community effect that represents deviation of community j's mean z-score from the state level mean, and 'k' is a random household effect that represents deviation of household jk's mean z-score from the jth community mean. The error terms σ_j and σ_{jk} are assumed to be normally distributed with zero mean and variances, $\sigma^2{}_c$ and $\sigma^{2,}{}_h$ respectively. As per the arguments above, these terms are non-zero and estimated by variance components models. To the extent that the greater homogeneity of within-cluster observations is not explained by the observed covariates, $\sigma^2_{h,}$ σ^2_{ct} will be larger (Gragnolati, 1999).

To evaluate the appropriateness of the multilevel models, I test whether the variances of the random part are different from zero over households and communities. The resulting estimates from the models can be used to assess the extent of contribution of different level to total before and after I have accounted for the observed effects of covariates x_{jk}. A significantly different amount from zero suggests appropriateness of random effect models (Marini and Gragnolati, 2006). The variance contributions of different levels are represented by the formulae:

$$c = \sigma^2 c /(\sigma^2 c + \sigma^2 h) \text{ for community level}$$

$$h = \sigma^2 h /(\sigma^2 c + \sigma^2 h) \text{ for household level}$$

Thus, the total variability in the individual HAZ scores can be divided into its two components; variance in children's nutritional status among households within communities, and variance among communities. By including covariates, the variance components models allow to examine the extent to which observed differences in the anthropometric scores are attributable to factors influencing variation at each level. The variance components model described above introduces a random intercept at each level assuming a constant effect of each of the covariates (on the outcome) across the clusters.

Hence, multilevel models are based on observations 14312 (NFHS I), 17447 (NFHS II), 16881 (NFHS III) approximately for each time point from households distributed in fifteen major states. Inclusion of separate levels for children and mothers are considered not necessary since 1:1 relationship is there with households.

DECOMPOSITION

I decompose Concentration Index into the contribution of each factor to asset and living standard related inequality in nutritional status where each contribution is a product of the sensitivity of stunting with respect to that factor and the degree of asset and living standard related inequality in that factor. STATA Version 11 is used for all the analyses.

EXPLANATORY VARIABLES HOUSEHOLD STANDARD OF LIVING AS THE PROXY FOR HOUSEHOLD ECONOMIC STATUS

Following the standard approach of assessing economic status of the household (Gwatkin *et al*., 2007). I use household assets, and different other living standard indicators provided commonly by the NFHS I, II and III. I prepare the household standard of living index based on different household characteristics and ownership of household assets using additive method following NFHS II valuation of assets and household characteristics. The items are type of house, toilet facility, drinking water, main fuel for cooking, ownership of agricultural land, irrigated land, livestock, has electricity or not, ownership of durables like tractor, thresher, water pump, bullock cart, sewing machine, fan, radio, refrigerator, television, motorcycle, car, bicycle, clock/watch. Then I divide the household SLI into three almost equal groups based on the scores.

Explanatory Variables Used as Controls

I chose other determinants of childhood under-nutrition based on the conceptual framework in the literature (UNICEF, 1990; Smith and Haddad, 1999; Gragnolati *et al.,* 2005; Svedberg, 2007; Kanjilal *et al.,* 2010). I consider certain individual characteristics of child as the proximate influencing factors of chronic under-nutrition. These predisposing factors include child's characteristics similar to other studies, such as, child's age in months in four categories

(0-5, 6-11, 12-23, 24-35 months), sex of the child (female, male), birth order (first, second, third or more), size of child at birth (large, average, small) as a proxy of birth weight (Som *et al.*, 2007), recommended feeding practice; denoted by exclusive breast feeding for infants below six months of age, introduction of complementary feeding along with or without breast milk at six months of age. In view of information provided by NFHS on child feeding, a child who eats any complementary food starting from 6 months of age irrespective of its breast feeding status is considered for latter feeding practice variable.

The controls on mother's characteristics include; education (illiterate, primary, secondary, higher), (Linnemayr *et al.*, 2008), employment status (employed or not) and place of birth for the child (child delivered at home or institution). On the household level, I include controls for household religion and ethnicity (Hindu and other minorities are two categories for religion, general and backward caste are two categories for ethnicity) since a large number of earlier studies found a significant linkage between scheduled tribe/scheduled caste households and childhood under-nutrition (Bawdekar and Ladusingh, 2008; Rajaram *et al.*, 2007). Community characteristic is regarded as the distant covariate of child under-nutrition in the model. This is believed to capture the heterogeneity through rural-urban place of residence keeping in mind the variation in childhood mortality and morbidity across rural and urban area.

RESULTS

Table 1 shows the descriptive statistics, Tables 2 and 3 show the percentage of stunted and concentration index values with their t statistics respectively. Tables 4 and 7 present the sample characteristics of fifteen major states in three time points and different state groups at 2005-06 respectively. Tables 5 and 8 present the stunting prevalence among children under the age of three in fifteen major states in three time points and different state groups

Table 1: Descriptive statistics

	Height for age z score	***Age of the child***	***Sex of the child***	***Birth order***	***Exclusive breast feeding***	***Complementary feeding***	***Size of the child at birth***	***Mother's education***	***Mother's employment status***	***Place of delivery***	***Standard of Living***	***Ethnicity***	***Religion***	***Location of residence***
N	48640	48640	48640	48640	48640	48640	48617	48581	48611	48632	48432	48023	48608	48640
Mean	–1.911	2.868	1.483	2.179	0.070	0.797	2.061	0.878	0.293	1.362	1.921	0.533	0.786	1.704
Median	–1.970	3.000	1.000	2.000	0.000	1.000	2.000	0.000	0.000	1.000	2.000	1.000	1.000	2.000
Standard deviation	1.788	1.039	0.500	0.838	0.256	0.402	0.624	1.018	0.455	0.481	0.795	0.499	0.410	0.457
Inter quartile range	2.250	2.000	1.000	2.000	0.000	0.000	0.000	2.000	1.000	1.000	2.000	1.000	0.000	1.000
Pseudo Standard Deviation	1.667	1.481	0.741	1.481	0.000	0.000	0.000	1.481	0.741	0.741	1.481	0.741	0.000	0.741
Skewness	0.429	–0.528	0.068	–0.347	3.364	–1.477	–0.043	0.619	0.911	0.574	0.141	–0.131	–1.391	–0.893
Kurtosis	3.741	2.103	1.005	1.510	12.319	3.182	2.554	1.921	1.830	1.329	1.595	1.017	2.935	1.798
Sum	–92938.1	139502.0	72133.0	106002.0	3415.0	38768.0	100203.0	42648.0	14229.0	66243.0	93057.0	25576.0	38182.0	82880.0
Range	12	3	1	2	1	1	2	3	1	1	2	1	1	1
Minimum	–6	1	1	1	0	0	1	0	0	1	1	0	0	1
Maximum	6	4	2	3	1	1	3	3	1	2	3	1	1	2

at 2005-06 respectively. The covariates included as controls in analytical models, with the primary aim of testing the degree of change in strength and magnitude of SLI over time in random intercept models are described in Table 6 (only model household is shown in the paper). For state groups all four models for each state group are shown with household and community as two clusters and also their contributions to total variance. The analysis is presented in the form of four models (Tables 9, 10, 11, 12): Null Model- the HAZ scores is the dependant variable with only SLI covariate included; Kid Model controls child specific predictors; Mother Model controls the mother-specific covariates. Household Model is the full model with all the model covariates at respective levels. These models are two-level random intercept models with the two clusters: household and community. Table 13 and Table 14 present variance component and decomposition results respectively.

Preliminary Finding

Table 2 related to preliminary findings describes the situation of different major Indian states with respect to chronic childhood under-nutrition. Prevalence of stunting was highest in Bihar and lowest in Kerala in 1992-93. In 1992-93, none of the states is showing prevalence below 30 percent. Maximum level was 60 percent. Three out of five children under the age of three were stunted in Bihar, Madhya Pradesh and Uttar Pradesh in that period. In Bihar and Madhya Pradesh the prevalence was reduced by only 2 to 3 percent in the next six to seven years. But, it reduced by 8 percent in another five to six years. However prevalence is still high. In Uttar Pradesh, Maharashtra, and Punjab the prevalence has not changed during nineties. It changed by eight to twelve percentage points in these states in the next five years except Maharashtra. In Maharashtra, the change is very slow like in Orissa, Gujarat, and Kerala. But status of undernourishment in Kerala is not comparable with the same in other three states as percentage of stunted below –2 Standard Deviation is already very low in Kerala

Table 2: Percentage of children under the age of three stunted in India by states (% below-2SD)

States	*1992-93*	*1998-99*	*2005-06*
Bihar	60.3	57.6	49.5
Madhya Pradesh	60	56.4	48
Uttar Pradesh	60	60.3	51.9
West Bengal	56.7	50.1	41.8
Assam	56.5	53.7	41.4
Orissa	50.8	49.1	43.9
Haryana	50.5	55.4	43.2
Gujarat	50.1	51.8	49.1
Karnataka	47.5	42	42.3
Maharashtra	47	47	43.9
Delhi	46.9	43.2	43.1
Himachal Pradesh	46.8	49	34.3
Rajasthan	45.5	59	40.1
Jammu & Kashmir	45.4	44.6	33
Punjab	45.2	45.2	34.6
North East	42.7	38.3	35.9
Andhra Pradesh	40.8	47.1	38.3
Tamil Nadu	40.8	35	31.1
Goa	34.8	21.8	25.8
Kerala	32.8	27.8	26.5

Source: NFHS rounds

compared to other states. In Karnataka, Delhi and Rajasthan prevalence is more or less 40 percent and there was approximately no change in the last ten years. In Andhra Pradesh and Haryana, percentage of stunted increased in first five years and then decreased by few percentage points in next five years. In West Bengal, Assam and Andhra Pradesh stunting percentage has fallen by more or equal to ten percentage points.

It is clear from Table 3 that, concentration of under-nutrition is higher among poor in all the states in all the time points. Over time, inequity in nutritional status between rich and poor are increasing. In Haryana, Orissa, Punjab inequity is increased in first decade of the millennium as compared to previous years. Rank of Kerala, Andhra Pradesh, Assam had drastic change between early and late nineties with respect to concentration of

Table 3: Concentration of undernourished children under the age of three in Indian states and their t statistics

States	*1992-93*	*t statistic*	*1998-99*	*t statistic*	*2005-06*	*t statistic*
Andhra Pradesh	–0.121	–1.56	–0.084	–1.35	–0.147	–3.18
Assam	–0.091	–1.06	–0.025	–5.51	–0.117	–2.66
Bihar	–0.040	–1.78	–0.046	–1.22	–0.069	–1.50
Delhi	–0.033	–0.75	–0.077	–4.08	–0.156	–2.32
Goa	–0.117	–1.71	–0.212	–3.11	–0.257	–13.33
Gujarat	–0.060	–4.69	–0.116	–1.58	–0.119	–2.88
Haryana	–0.050	–2.75	–0.078	–2.58	–0.155	–3.02
Himachal	–0.036	–1.49	–0.072	–1.85	–0.127	–2.72
Jammu & Kashmir	–0.090	–3.18	–0.132	–1.68	–0.173	–3.95
Karnataka	–0.088	–1.54	–0.111	–1.46	–0.128	–2.38
Kerala	–0.143	–3.25	–0.099	–2.16	–0.128	–1.57
Madhya Pradesh	–0.035	–1.64	–0.068	–1.38	–0.047	–1.37
Maharashtra	–0.088	–4.30	–0.117	–2.20	–0.145	–2.96
North East	–0.057	–2.01	–0.100	–1.47	–0.121	–2.43
Orissa	–0.047	–1.53	–0.091	–1.43	–0.198	–2.78
Punjab	0.047	–2.31	–0.110	–5.81	–0.233	–3.77
Rajasthan	0.000	0.05	–0.060	–1.38	–0.115	–2.65
Tamil Nadu	–0.121	–1.68	–0.132	–1.48	–0.138	–2.19
Uttar Pradesh	–0.035	–1.64	–0.061	–1.28	–0.115	–2.51
West Bengal	–0.048	–1.72	–0.141	–1.87	–0.138	–2.30

undernourishment. The situation got better in next period. However, inequity increased after that period.

Comparing the sample characteristics of NFHS I, II and III in Table 4; it is clear that number of children are almost selected in equal percentage from each socioeconomic group in NFHS III than NFHS I or NFHS II. If I disaggregate by age, information is available in higher percentage for more than one year old children. Sample contains more boys than girls which are also reflected in the sex ratio of India (CENSUS, 2001). Most of the households have three or more number of children though the percentage gradually reduced over time. Near about 60 percent of children were born with average size at birth. Among children aged 0-5 months, near about 40 percent are exclusively breastfed and the percentage

Table 4: Sample characteristics NFHS I, NFHS II and NFHS III

	NFHS I		***NFHS II***		***NFHS III***	
	N	***%***	***N***	***%***	***N***	***%***
Standard of Living						
Poor	5,305	37.1	5,942	34.5	6,113	36.2
Middle	3,984	27.9	8,153	47.3	5,382	31.9
Rich	5,017	35.1	3,153	18.3	5,383	31.9
Child's characteristics						
Age						
0-5 months	2,229	15.6	2,774	15.9	2,214	13.1
6-11 months	2,375	16.6	2,935	16.8	2,931	17.4
12-23 months	5,183	36.2	5,905	33.9	5,837	34.6
24-35 months	4,525	31.6	5,833	33.4	5,899	34.9
Sex						
Boy	7,258	50.7	9,055	51.9	8,834	52.3
Girl	7,054	49.3	8,392	48.1	8,047	47.7
Birth order						
First	3,576	25.0	4,691	26.9	5,227	31.0
Second	3,417	23.9	4,618	26.5	4,895	29.0
Third and more	7,319	51.1	8,138	46.6	6,759	40.0
Size of the child at birth						
Large	1,852	13.0	2,563	14.7	3,649	21.6
Average	9,402	65.7	10,621	60.9	9,497	56.3
Small	3,048	21.3	4,253	24.4	3,732	22.1
Child feeding practice						
Not exclusively breastfed for 0-5 months	1,303	58.5	1,527	55.1	1,262	57.0
Exclusively breastfed for 0-5 months	926	41.5	1,247	45.0	952	43.0
Not introduced complementary feeding at the age of 6 months	3,880	32.1	2,140	14.6	639	4.4
Introduced complementary feeding at the age of 6 months	8,203	67.9	12,533	85.4	14028	95.6
Mother's characteristics						
Mother's education						
Illiterate Mother	8,857	62.1	9,287	53.3	7,188	42.6
Educated up to primary	2,023	14.2	2,718	15.6	2,299	13.6

Table 4: *(Contd...)*

Table 4: (*Contd...*)

	NFHS I		*NFHS II*		*NFHS III*	
	N	*%*	*N*	*%*	*N*	*%*
Educated up to secondary	2,917	20.5	3,996	22.9	6,106	36.2
Has higher education	462	3.2	1,440	8.3	1,288	7.6
Mother's employment status						
Unemployed	10,803	75.6	12,130	69.5	11449	67.8
Employed	3,484	24.4	5,315	30.5	5430	32.2
Health service use						
Child delivered at home	10,608	74.1	11,260	64.6	9,153	54.2
Child delivered at institution household characteristics	3,701	25.9	6,183	35.5	7,727	45.8
Religion						
Hindu	11,119	77.7	14,072	80.7	12,991	77.0
Muslim & other minorities	3,193	22.3	3,361	19.3	3,872	23.0
Caste						
Forward caste	11,192	78.2	6,310	36.4	4,945	30.2
Backward caste	3,120	21.8	11,011	63.6	11,445	69.8
Location						
Urban	3,545	24.8	4,649	26.7	6,206	36.8
Rural	10,767	75.2	12,798	73.4	10,675	63.2

changed marginally over time. But for children aged 6 to 35 months introduction of complementary feeding in timely manner is visible for 68 percent in 1992-93, 85 percent in 1998-99 and 96 percent in 2005-06. Thus it may be an indicator that feeding practice of older children improved substantially, though the same for younger children is far behind. Over time it is also visible that mother's educational status has improved over time. In 1992-93, near about 62 percent mothers were illiterate; such percentage reduced by 9 percentage points in 1998-99 and by 10 percentage points in 2005-06. Over time female labour force participation has increased. Near about 80 percent children belong to Hindu families. There is a difference in percentage of ethnic population in the sample in NFHS I, NFHS II and NFHS III. In NFHS I, only 22 percent children were from backward community, while it covered 64 percent (NFHS II) and 70 percent (NFHS III) in later surveys. Three out of five children are from rural India. Over time percentage of home delivery reduced. Side by side sample contains more urban respondents with time.

Table 5 shows pattern of prevalence in three time points by background characteristics of children under the age of three in fifteen major states. Over time prevalence of stunting has been reduced among children with different standard of living. However decline in stunting percentage is highest in richer families, then in middle class families and lowest reduction is experienced by poor families. Prevalence is all time higher among poor children.

Table 5: Prevalence of stunting by different factors as per conceptual framework NFHS I, NFHS II and NFHS III

	NFHS I		*NFHS II*		*NFHS III*	
	N	*%*	*N*	*%*	*N*	*%*
Standard of Living						
Poor	3,107	58.6	3,580	60.3	3,253	53.2
Middle	2,229	56.0	4,294	52.7	2,473	46.0
Rich	2,163	43.1	1,110	35.2	1,617	30.0
Child's characteristics						
Age						
0-5 months	602	27.0	751	27.1	467	21.1
6-11 months	914	38.5	1,036	35.3	780	26.6
12-23 months	2,958	57.1	3,478	58.9	2,973	50.9
24-35 months	3,029	66.9	3,837	65.8	3,124	53.0
Sex						
Boy	3,940	54.3	4,712	52.0	3,957	44.8
Girl	3,563	50.5	4,390	52.3	3,387	42.1
Birth order						
First	1,738	48.6	2,174	46.3	1,950	37.3
Second	1,682	49.2	2,261	49.0	2,024	41.4
Third and more	4,083	55.8	4,667	57.4	3,370	49.9
Size of the child at birth						
Large	825	44.6	1,142	44.6	1,468	40.2
Average	4,945	52.6	5,435	51.2	3,989	42.0
Small	1,726	56.6	2,520	59.3	1,886	50.5

Table 5: (*Contd...*)

Table 5: (*Contd...*)

	NFHS I		*NFHS II*		*NFHS III*	
	N	%	*N*	%	*N*	%
Child feeding practice						
Not exclusively breastfed for 0-5 months	333	25.6	411	26.9	251	19.9
Exclusively breastfed for 0-5 months	269	29.1	340	27.3	216	22.7
Not introduced complementary feeding at the age of 6 months	2,258	58.2	1337	62.5	349	54.6
Introduced complementary feeding at the age of 6 months	4,643	56.6	7,014	56.0	6,528	46.5
Mother's characteristics						
Mother's education						
Illiterate Mother	5,182	58.5	5,631	60.6	3,830	53.3
Educated up to primary	1,038	51.3	1,419	52.2	1,070	46.5
Educated up to secondary	1,131	38.8	1,649	41.3	2,196	36.0
Has higher education	122	26.4	399	27.7	248	19.3
Mother's employment status						
Employed	1,990	57.1	3,136	59.0	2,755	50.7
Unemployed	5,498	50.9	5,965	49.2	4,587	40.1
Health service use						
Child delivered at home	6,021	56.8	6,595	58.6	4,705	51.4
Child delivered at institution	1,480	40.0	2,505	40.5	2,639	34.2
Household characteristics						
Religion						
Hindu	5,869	52.8	7,403	52.6	5,696	43.9
Muslim & other minorities	1,634	51.2	1,688	50.2	1,635	42.2
Caste						
Forward caste	5,760	51.5	2,977	47.2	1,770	35.8
Backward caste	1,743	55.9	6,049	54.9	5,367	46.9
Location						
Urban	1,629	46.0	1,949	41.9	2,279	36.7
Rural	5,874	54.6	7,153	55.9	5,065	47.5
Total	7,496	52.4	9,102	52.2	7,344	43.5

Among children under the age group of five months, rate of reduction in stunting is lowest. Surprisingly, weaning period children – most of the stunted comes from that group – have experienced highest fall though the rate of falling is not much higher. On average, boys are always more stunted than girls. Stunting prevalence is consistently higher with higher birth order, smaller size at birth, children with poor dietary intake, children of illiterate mothers, employed mothers, who delivered at home, belong to backward communities and lives in rural area. Over time gap in prevalence has been increased between backward-forward caste and rural-urban area with improvement among forward caste and urban children.

It is evident from Table 6 that, children with lower living standard, older age, sex being male, higher birth order, smaller size, not started complementary feeding at 6th month of age, children of illiterate or less educated mother, employed mother, mother with less contact to health services, children belonging to backward class and living in rural area are more undernourished. Over time, marginal impact of medium and higher SLI compared to lower SLI has increased. Similar pattern is visible with respect to child's age, number of children, child's complementary feeding practice, mother's employment, gender and social position. But spatial inequity, inequity with respect to mother's education and health seeking is reduced for stunting prevalence. Pattern of marginal impact has linearly changed for children of medium SLI, backward social group or exclusively breastfed children. Non-linear movement is visible for children belonging to higher SLI, different age group, male children, children of smaller size, complementary feeding practice, mother's education, employment status, contact with health service and location of residence.

PATTERN OF INEQUITY IN NUTRITIONAL STATUS ACROSS STATES IN ONE TIME POINT

Table 7 shows sample characteristics by different state groups. In the sample of HPHI state 60 percent of sample children belong to

Table 6: Random intercept model with PSU and household level variation in mean z score showing socioeconomic gradient with and without controlling for household and PSU level attributes in three time points

	NFHS I	*NFHS II*	*NFHS III*
Low standard of living (Ref.)			
Medium standard of living	0.063*	0.060**	0.116***
SE	0.037	0.029	0.033
High standard of living	0.320***	0.307***	0.401***
SE	0.041	0.044	0.041
0-5 months (Ref.)			
6-11 months	–0.556***	–0.476***	–0.522***
SE	0.054	0.049	0.052
12-23 months	–1.236***	–1.355***	–1.425***
SE	0.050	0.045	0.048
24-35 months	–1.648***	–1.703***	–1.502***
SE	0.053	0.046	0.048
Male child (Ref.)			
Sex of the child (Female)	0.174***	0.061**	0.114***
SE	0.027	0.024	0.024
1st Birth order (Ref.)			
2nd Birth order	0.009	–0.031	-0.044
SE	0.039	0.033	0.031
3rd and more	–0.075**	–0.094***	–0.094***
SE	0.035	0.032	0.033
Size of the child - Large (Ref.)			
Average	–0.313***	–0.238***	–0.067**
SE	0.043	0.036	0.032
Small	–0.517***	–0.541***	–0.341***
SE	0.050	0.041	0.038
Not exclusively breastfed children (0-5 months) (Ref.)			
Exclusively breastfed children (0-5 months)	–0.016	0.146**	0.186**
SE	0.074	0.069	0.088
Children not introduced complementary feeding at 6 months (Ref.)			
Children with any complementary feeding at 6 months	–0.037	0.005	0.279***
SE	0.035	0.040	0.068

Table 6: (*Contd...*)

Table 6: (*Contd...*)

	NFHS I	*NFHS II*	*NFHS III*
Respondent is illiterate (Ref.)			
Educated up to Primary	0.150***	0.194***	0.082**
SE	0.044	0.037	0.041
Educated up to Secondary	0.353***	0.400***	0.252***
SE	0.046	0.037	0.036
Has higher education	0.589***	0.652***	0.621***
SE	0.094	0.057	0.061
Respondent is unemployed (Ref.)			
Respondent is employed	–0.043	0.011	–0.110***
SE	0.037	0.029	0.030
Child delivered at home (Ref.)			
Child delivered at institution	0.212***	0.278***	0.200***
SE	0.041	0.031	0.032
Child belong to minorities (Ref.)			
Hindu	0.021	–0.004	0.038
SE	0.041	0.034	0.035
General (Ref.)			
Backward caste	–0.014	–0.110***	–0.147***
SE	0.039	0.028	0.031
Lives in urban area (Ref.)			
Lives in rural area	0.008	–0.174***	–0.035
SE	0.050	0.034	0.035
Intercept	–1.137***	–0.871	–1.092
SE	0.100	0.090	0.107
Number of observations	14216	17094	16366
Wald chi^2	2395.470	4293.570	3308.03
P>chi^2	0.0000	0.0000	0.0000
Log likelihood	-27375.971	–32249.414	–30651.795

Significance level: * p<.1; ** p<.05; *** p<.01

poor socioeconomic group. HPLI states also have higher percentage of children in poor SLI group. In other two state groups middle to higher economic group percentage is higher (though in a particular state group this may not be distributed uniformly across all the members). Regarding children disaggregated by age group shows that almost 70 percent of children of each state group belongs to 12-35 months age group. In all the state groups except Orissa, proportion of male children is higher than female children. About

Table 7: Sample characteristics of the child population under the age of three in different state groups in 2005-06

	HPHI		***HPMI***		***HPLI***		***MPHI***	
	N	***%***	***N***	***%***	***N***	***%***	***N***	***%***
Standard of Living								
Poor	494	60.2	758	23.4	3,905	44.2	956	24.0
Middle	195	23.8	1,286	39.7	2,658	30.1	1,243	31.3
Rich	131	16.0	1,198	37.0	2,277	25.8	1,777	44.7
Child's characteristics								
Age								
0-5 months	116	14.1	303	9.3	1,324	15.0	471	11.9
6-11 months	140	17.0	591	18.2	1,529	17.3	671	16.9
12-23 months	288	35.0	1,151	35.5	2,979	33.7	1,419	35.7
24-35 months	278	33.8	1,198	36.9	3,008	34.0	1,415	35.6
Sex								
Girl	415	50.5	1,520	46.9	4,257	48.2	1,855	46.7
Boy	407	49.5	1,723	53.1	4,583	51.8	2,121	53.4
Birth order								
First	261	31.8	1,180	36.4	2,291	25.9	1,495	37.6
Second	242	29.4	1,151	35.5	2,163	24.5	1,339	33.7
Third and more	319	38.8	912	28.1	4,386	49.6	1,142	28.7
Size of the child at birth								
Large	188	22.9	1,048	32.4	1,565	17.7	848	21.3
Average	391	47.6	1,543	47.6	5,320	60.2	2,243	56.4
Small	243	29.6	649	20.0	1,955	22.1	885	22.3
Child feeding practice								
Not exclusively breastfed for 0-5 months	54	46.6	179	59.1	767	57.9	262	55.6
Exclusively breastfed for 0-5 months	62	53.5	124	40.9	557	42.1	209	44.4
Not introduced complementary feeding at the age of 6 months	40	5.7	108	3.7	767	57.9	143	4.1
Introduced complementary feeding at the age of 6 months	666	94.3	2,832	96.3	557	42.1	3,362	95.9
Mother's characteristics								
Mother's education								
Illiterate Mother	351	42.7	907	28.0	4,875	55.2	1,055	26.5
Educated up to primary	154	18.7	477	14.7	1,163	13.2	505	12.7

Table 7: *(Contd...)*

Table 7: (*Contd...*)

	HPHI		*HPMI*		*HPLI*		*MPHI*	
	N	*%*	*N*	*%*	*N*	*%*	*N*	*%*
Educated up to secondary	286	34.8	1,592	49.1	2,221	25.1	2,007	50.5
Has higher education	31	3.8	267	8.2	581	6.6	409	10.3
Mother's employment status								
Employed	223	27.1	995	30.7	3,352	37.9	860	21.6
Unemployed	599	72.9	2,247	69.3	5,487	62.1	3,116	78.4
Health service use								
Child delivered at home	483	58.8	863	26.6	6,283	71.1	1,524	38.3
Child delivered at institution	339	41.2	2,379	73.4	2,557	28.9	2,452	61.7
Household characteristics								
Religion								
Hindu	781	95.7	2,649	81.7	7,036	79.7	2,525	63.5
Muslim & other minorities	35	4.3	592	18.3	1,794	20.3	1,451	36.5
Caste								
Forward caste	235	28.9	718	22.3	2,069	24.0	1,923	51.7
Backward caste	577	71.1	2,505	77.7	6,565	76.0	1,798	48.3
Location								
Urban	202	24.6	1,577	48.6	2,727	30.9	1,700	42.8
Rural	620	75.4	1,666	51.4	6,113	69.2	2,276	57.2

40 percent children in Orissa and 50 percent children in HPLI states are of three to higher birth order compared to other two state groups (approximately 28 percent). Regarding size of the child at birth majority born with average size. Except Orissa, almost 3 out of 5 children are not exclusively breastfed in the age group of 0-5 months. In relation to timely initiation of complementary food more than 90 percent was started with it at 6th month except HPLI states (42 percent). Higher percentage of illiterate mothers lives in HPHI and HPLI states; near about 70 percent mothers are unemployed in all the major states. In HPLI states 70 percent of delivery is home delivery which is 60 percent in Orissa. The scenario is reverse in other two groups. Sixty to ninety percent of children belong to Hindu families. Along with it, except MPHI states, 3 to 4 out of 5 children belong to backward communities in other states.

Table 8 describes the prevalence of stunting among children under the age of three in different state groups in 2005-06. It is evident that children of poor socioeconomic group in HPHI state show highest prevalence across different state groups. Next are children in HPLI and MPHI states. HPLI states show highest prevalence among weaning period children followed by HPHI state which also visible in relation to introduction of complementary feeding. In other words, children who introduced complementary feeding after 6 months of age are more stunted and the prevalence is higher in HPHI and HPLI states. Stunting is higher among children who are delivered at home in almost all the states. Higher prevalence is observed among children of illiterate mothers,

Table 8: Stunting prevalence of the child population under the age of three in different state groups

	HPHI		*HPMI*		*HPLI*		*MPHI*	
	N	*%*	*N*	*%*	*N*	*%*	*N*	*%*
Standard of Living								
Poor	272	55.1	371	48.9	2,099	53.8	511	53.5
Middle	71	36.4	553	43.0	1,308	49.2	541	43.5
Rich	25	19.1	344	28.7	751	33.0	497	28.0
Child's characteristics								
Age								
0-5 months	35	30.2	53	17.5	289	21.8	90	19.1
6-11 months	42	30.0	145	24.5	437	28.6	156	23.3
12-23 months	147	51.0	506	44.0	1,662	55.8	658	46.4
24-35 months	145	52.2	564	47.1	1,770	58.8	645	45.6
Sex								
Girl	187	45.1	570	37.5	1,939	45.6	691	37.3
Boy	182	44.7	698	40.5	2,219	48.4	858	40.5
Birth order								
First	96	36.8	400	33.9	938	40.9	516	34.5
Second	105	43.4	436	37.9	970	44.9	513	38.3
Third and more	168	52.7	432	47.4	2,250	51.3	520	45.5
Size of the child at birth								
Large	67	35.6	389	37.1	707	45.2	305	36.0
Average	173	44.3	569	36.9	2,426	45.6	821	36.6
Small	129	53.1	309	47.6	1,025	52.4	423	47.8

Table 8: *(Contd...)*

Table 8: (*Contd...*)

	HPHI		*HPMI*		*HPLI*		*MPHI*	
	N	***%***	***N***	***%***	***N***	***%***	***N***	***%***
Child feeding practice								
Not exclusively breastfed for 0-5 months	17	31.5	26	14.5	159	20.7	49	18.7
Exclusively breastfed for 0-5 months	18	29.0	27	21.8	130	23.3	41	19.6
Not introduced complementary feeding at the age of 6 months	24	60.0	49	45.4	207	59.5	69	48.3
Introduced complementary feeding at the age of 6 months	310	46.6	1,166	41.2	3,662	51.1	1,390	41.3
Mother's characteristics								
Mother's education								
Illiterate Mother	206	58.7	462	50.9	2,610	53.5	552	52.3
Educated up to primary	77	50.0	208	43.6	557	47.9	228	45.2
Educated up to secondary	82	28.7	547	34.4	877	39.5	690	34.4
Has higher education	4	12.9	51	19.1	114	19.6	79	19.3
Mother's employment status								
Employed	128	57.4	485	48.7	1,760	52.5	382	44.4
Unemployed	241	40.2	782	34.8	2,397	43.7	1,167	37.5
Health service use								
Child delivered at home	258	53.4	444	51.5	3,254	51.8	749	49.2
Child delivered at institution	111	32.7	824	34.6	904	35.4	800	32.6
Household characteristics								
Religion								
Hindu	345	44.17	1,067	40.3	3,280	46.6	1,004	39.8
Muslim & other minorities	21	60	199	33.6	870	48.5	545	37.6
Caste								
Forward caste	77	32.8	233	32.5	783	37.8	677	35.2
Backward caste	287	49.7	1,030	41.1	3,275	49.9	775	43.1
Location								
Urban	79	39.1	521	33.0	1,075	39.4	604	35.5
Rural	290	46.8	747	44.8	3,083	50.4	945	41.5
Total	368	44.9	1,268	39.1	4,158	47.0	1,549	39.0

employed mothers, children of backward communities and minor groups and the percentage is higher in HPHI and HPLI states. Rural children of almost all the states are suffering more in higher percentage.

From Table 9, it is evident that, in HPHI state Orissa, children belonging to middle or high SLI group have higher z score than

Table 9: Random intercept models with different levels of controls with two clusters - village/town and household in High Prevalent High Inequity state in 2005-06

NFHS 3	*Model Null*	*Model Kid*	*Model Mother*	*Model Household*
Low standard of living (Ref.)				
Medium standard of living	0.669***	0.609***	0.461***	0.450***
SE	0.138	0.139	0.146	0.15
High standard of living	1.011***	0.907***	0.454**	0.463**
SE	0.167	0.171	0.2	0.21
0-5 months (Ref.)				
6-11 months		0.103	0.103	0.121
SE		0.23	0.228	0.232
12-23 months		–0.629***	–0.586***	–0.545**
SE		0.219	0.218	0.222
24-35 months		–0.711***	–0.672***	–0.621***
SE		0.217	0.217	0.222
Male child (Ref.)				
Sex of the child (Female)		–0.074	–0.09	–0.075
SE		0.108	0.108	0.11
1st Birth order (Ref.)				
2nd Birth order		–0.103	–0.062	–0.062
SE		0.137	0.138	0.141
3rd and more		–0.189	–0.04	–0.036
SE		0.134	0.143	0.146
Size of the child – Large (Ref.)				
Average		–0.096	–0.076	–0.09
SE		0.141	0.14	0.143
Small		–0.439***	–0.420***	–0.427***
SE		0.154	0.153	0.154
Not exclusively breastfed children (0-5 months) (Ref.)				

Table 9: (*Contd...*)

Table 9: (*Contd...*)

NFHS 3	*Model Null*	*Model Kid*	*Model Mother*	*Model Household*
Exclusively breastfed children (0-5 months)		0.594	0.556	0.54
SE		0.368	0.369	0.372
Children not introduced complementary feeding at 6 months (Ref.)				
Children introduced any complementary feeding at 6 months		0.461	0.417	0.396
SE		0.29	0.289	0.291
Respondent is illiterate (Ref.)				
Educated up to Primary			0.039	0.011
SE			0.161	0.164
Educated up to Secondary			0.452***	0.399**
SE			0.162	0.167
Has higher education			1.429***	1.319***
SE			0.341	0.349
Respondent is unemployed (Ref.)				
Respondent is employed			–0.112	–0.118
SE			0.138	0.141
Child delivered at home (Ref.)				
Child delivered at institution			–0.023	–0.017
SE			0.132	0.135
Child belongs to minorities (Ref.)				
Hindu				0.292
SE				0.293
General (Ref.)				
Backward caste				–0.138
SE				0.144
Lives in urban area (Ref.)				
Lives in rural area				0.054
SE				0.172
Intercept	–1.99***	–1.577***	–1.697***	–1.926***
SE	0.0836	0.417	0.423	0.534
Number of observations	820	820	820	805
Wald Chi^2	47.84	108.44	133.03	126.91
P value>Chi^2	0.0000	0.0000	0.0000	0.0000
Log Likelihood	–1542.1699	–1526.7281	–1520.2885	–1496.5251

Significance level: * p<.1; ** p<.05; *** p<.01

poor children. Children have lower z score with older age, higher birth order, smaller size at birth. Controlling for child level traits reduces the influence of socioeconomic status. In other words, impact of socioeconomic disparity works through child characteristics related disparities. Controlling mother's attributes further reduces the impact of socioeconomic status as it works through the mother's educational achievement. Children of illiterate or less educated mothers are undernourished. Though household factors are not significant, socioeconomic status is working through the social status of households.

In HPMI states, children belonging to poorer families, older in age compared to the children under six months of age, girls, children of 3rd or higher birth order, smaller size at birth, not introduced with complementary feeding at the age of six months, illiterate mothers, mothers work outside home and child is delivered at home – such children are more undernourished (Table 10). In HPMI states number of children, feeding practice and access to health care are additionally significant compared to HPHI state in India. In model null, higher stunting among poor children compared to children belonging to middle or rich SLI group and it is highly significant. Controlling of child attributes shows that these factors were confounding the impact of socioeconomic status. Then controlling mother's traits along with children's features; it is evident that mother level factors are also confounding the impact of socioeconomic status. Though household level factors are not significant influencing ones, it is obvious that impact of socioeconomic status is working through the household's social status.

In HPLI states, model null shows that poor children are more undernourished (Table 11). Controlling child characteristics shows that heterogeneity in nutritional status by socioeconomic group is partly explained by child's characteristics- children with higher age, higher birth order, smaller size at birth, and for whom, timely initiation of complementary feeding is not done are more stunted. Impact of socioeconomic status is further explained through

Table 10: Random intercept models with different levels of controls with two clusters - village/town and household in High Prevalent Moderate Inequity states in 2005-06

NFHS 3	*Model Null*	*Model Kid*	*Model Mother*	*Model Household*
Low standard of living (Ref.)				
Medium standard of living	0.206**	0.178**	0.089	0.057
SE	0.082	0.080	0.081	0.083
High standard of living	0.688***	0.602***	0.365***	0.323***
SE	0.086	0.085	0.091	0.095
0-5 months (Ref.)				
6-11 months		–0.461***	–0.446***	–0.434***
SE		0.131	0.130	0.131
12-23 months		–1.304***	–1.282***	–1.270***
SE		0.125	0.124	0.125
24-35 months		–1.361***	–1.296***	–1.285***
SE		0.123	0.123	0.124
Male child (Ref.)				
Sex of the child (Female)		0.095*	0.095*	0.090
SE		0.056	0.056	0.056
1st Birth order (Ref.)				
2nd Birth order		–0.096	–0.047	–0.051
SE		0.065	0.065	0.065
3rd and more		–0.315***	–0.169**	–0.178**
SE		0.074	0.076	0.077
Size of the child – Large (Ref.)				
Average		–0.006	–0.021	–0.015
SE		0.067	0.067	0.067
Small		–0.357***	–0.343***	–0.326***
SE		0.084	0.083	0.084
Not exclusively breastfed children (0-5 months) (Ref.)				
Exclusively breastfed children (0-5 months)		0.231	0.214	0.259
SE		0.225	0.225	0.226
Children not introduced complementary feeding at 6 months (Ref.)				
Children with any complementary feeding at 6 months		0.340**	0.323*	0.323*

Table 10: (*Contd...*)

Table 10: (*Contd...*)

NFHS 3	*Model Null*	*Model Kid*	*Model Mother*	*Model Household*
SE		0.169	0.168	0.168
Respondent is illiterate (Ref.)				
Educated up to Primary			0.078	0.074
SE			0.097	0.097
Educated up to Secondary			0.265***	0.249***
SE			0.082	0.082
Has higher education			0.636***	0.591***
SE			0.133	0.134
Respondent is unemployed (Ref.)				
Respondent is employed			–0.238***	–0.209***
SE			0.070	0.071
Child delivered at home (Ref.)				
Child delivered at institution			0.176**	0.157**
SE			0.075	0.076
Child belongs to minorities (Ref.)				
Hindu				–0.059
SE				0.089
General (Ref.)				
Backward caste				–0.066
SE				0.082
Lives in urban area (Ref.)				
Lives in rural area				–0.100
SE				0.079
Intercept	–1.769	–0.943	–1.146	–0.956
SE	0.068	0.233	0.240	0.264
Number of observations	3242	3239	3238	3217
Wald Chi^2	75.34	416.39	480.96	473.79
P value>Chi^2	0.0000	0.0000	0.0000	0.0000
Log Likelihood	–6333.9293	–6188.0800	–6165.9129	–6131.1342

Significance level: * p<.1; ** p<.05; *** p<.01

mother's characteristics - children of illiterate or less educated mother, employed mother and children delivered at home are more stunted. Controlling of household characteristics shows less direct impact of economic status which is coming through the social position of the household. Children belonging to Muslim communities, Scheduled Caste or Scheduled Tribe or other backward communities are more undernourished.

Table 11: Random intercept models with different levels of controls with two clusters - village/town and household in High Prevalent Low Inequity states in 2005-06

NFHS 3	*Model Null*	*Model Kid*	*Model Mother*	*Model Household*
Low standard of living (Ref.)				
Medium standard of living	0.229***	0.189***	0.127***	0.098**
SE	0.045	0.043	0.044	0.045
High Standard of living	0.794***	0.712***	0.405***	0.354***
SE	0.049	0.048	0.056	0.058
0-5 months (Ref.)				
6-11 months		–0.643***	–0.637***	–0.626***
SE		0.069	0.068	0.069
12-23 months		–1.605***	–1.588***	–1.586***
SE		0.063	0.063	0.064
24-35 months		–1.739***	–1.721***	–1.726***
SE		0.063	0.063	0.063
Male child (Ref.)				
Sex of the child (Female)		0.131***	0.136***	0.135***
SE		0.034	0.034	0.034
1st Birth order (Ref.)				
2nd Birth order		–0.092**	–0.053	–0.077
SE		0.047	0.047	0.047
3rd and more		–0.189***	–0.051	–0.067
SE		0.043	0.044	0.045
Size of the child – Large (Ref.)				
Average		–0.039	–0.026	–0.030
SE		0.047	0.047	0.048
Small		–0.293***	–0.269***	–0.278***
SE		0.056	0.055	0.056
Not exclusively breastfed children (0-5 months) (Ref.)				
Exclusively breastfed children (0-5 months)		0.135	0.124	0.124
SE		0.118	0.118	0.119
Children not introduced complementary feeding at 6 months (Ref.)				
Children with any complementary feeding at 6 months		0.314***	0.276***	0.265***

Table 11: (*Contd...*)

Table 11: (*Contd...*)

NFHS 3	*Model Null*	*Model Kid*	*Model Mother*	*Model Household*
SE		0.092	0.091	0.092
Respondent is illiterate (Ref.)				
Educated up to Primary			0.110**	0.093*
SE			0.055	0.056
Educated up to Secondary			0.271***	0.235***
SE			0.050	0.051
Has higher education			0.686***	0.593***
SE			0.088	0.091
Respondent is unemployed (Ref.)				
Respondent is employed			–0.135***	–0.112***
SE			0.039	0.041
Child delivered at home (Ref.)				
Child delivered at institution			0.188***	0.161***
SE			0.046	0.047
Child belongs to minorities (Ref.)				
Hindu				0.109**
SE				0.053
General (Ref.)				
Backward caste				–0.211***
SE				0.048
Lives in urban area (Ref.)				
Lives in rural area				–0.086
SE				0.054
Intercept	–2.074	–1.072	–1.188	–0.989
SE	0.032	0.130	0.132	0.149
Number of observations	8840	8840	8839	8623
Wald Chi^2	262.79	1838.49	1990.41	1984.51
P value>Chi^2	0.0000	0.0000	0.0000	0.0000
Log Likelihood	–17407.9800	–16738.4160	–16683.5930	–16276.6320

Significance level: * p<.1; ** p<.05; *** p<.01

In MPHI states also socioeconomic gradient of stunting is highly significant like other states (Table 12). Similar to before, controlling of child attributes shows that impact of socioeconomic status has been decreased and child's age, sex, birth order and size are highly significant influencing factors. Children of higher age, boys, children of higher birth order, and smaller size are more undernourished. However, the fact is that one causal pathway of

Table 12: Random intercept models with different levels of controls with two clusters - village/town and household in Moderate Prevalent High Inequity states in 2005-06

NFHS 3	*Model Null*	*Model Kid*	*Model Mother*	*Model Household*
Low standard of living (Ref.)				
Medium standard of living	0.248***	0.224***	0.128*	0.158**
SE	0.069	0.067	0.069	0.074
High standard of living	0.860***	0.775***	0.529***	0.576***
SE	0.065	0.065	0.075	0.080
0-5 months (Ref.)				
6-11 months		–0.282***	–0.285***	–0.382***
SE		0.104	0.103	0.107
12-23 months		–1.200***	–1.187***	–1.257***
SE		0.097	0.097	0.100
24-35 months		–1.212***	–1.199***	–1.245***
SE		0.096	0.096	0.099
Male child (Ref.)				
Sex of the child (Female)		0.118**	0.127**	0.110**
SE		0.047	0.047	0.048
1st Birth order (Ref.)				
2nd Birth order		–0.042	0.005	0.019
SE		0.055	0.055	0.057
3rd and more		–0.201***	–.073	–0.086
SE		0.060	0.064	0.066
Size of the child – Large (Ref.)				
Average		–0.132**	–0.131**	–0.127**
SE		0.061	0.060	0.063
Small		–0.465***	–0.425***	–0.416***
SE		0.072	0.072	0.075
Not exclusively breastfed children (0-5 months) (Ref.)				
Exclusively breastfed children (0-5 months)		0.268	0.252	0.216
SE		0.177	0.177	0.181
Children not introduced complementary feeding at 6 months (Ref.)				
Children with any complementary feeding at 6 months		0.186	0.151	0.161

Table 12: (*Contd...*)

Table 12: (*Contd...*)

NFHS 3	*Model Null*	*Model Kid*	*Model Mother*	*Model Household*
SE		0.134	0.133	0.136
Respondent is illiterate (Ref.)				
Educated up to Primary			0.021	–0.008
SE			0.084	0.089
Educated up to Secondary			0.172**	0.148**
SE			0.072	0.074
Has higher education			0.557***	0.541***
SE			0.108	0.112
Respondent is unemployed (Ref.)				
Respondent is employed			–0.002	0.006
SE			0.060	0.062
Child delivered at home (Ref.)				
Child delivered at institution			0.206***	0.203***
SE			0.058	0.061
Child belongs to minorities (Ref.)				
Hindu				–0.028
SE				0.056
General (Ref.)				
Backward caste				–0.141***
SE				0.052
Lives in urban area (Ref.)				
Lives in rural area				0.104*
SE				0.058
Intercept	–1.968	–1.118	–1.305	–1.232
SE	0.053	0.187	0.191	0.208
Number of observations	3976	3976	3976	3721
Wald Chi^2	207.64	729.78	793.44	750.55
P value>Chi^2	0.0000	0.0000	0.0000	0.0000
Log Likelihood	–7428.9998	–7219.7454	–7202.0506	–6740.5645

Significance level: * p<.1; ** p<.05; *** p<.01

socioeconomic status is child's characteristics. When mother related traits are controlled the magnitude of impact of socioeconomic status again decreased. Children of illiterate or less educated mothers and who seek less or no health care from health facility are more stunted. Household's social status and place of residence act as confounders to socioeconomic gradient of chronic under-nutrition as controlling of such factors increases the magnitude of impact of socioeconomic status.

VARIANCE COMPONENTS

Table 13 represents variance components results. In almost all the major states, heterogeneity among children controlling for child, mother and household characteristics are more between households rather than between two communities since community level variation is lower than household level variations. However, controlling for child, maternal, household and community characteristics, the higher household level variation reconfirms that a child from richer family possesses different nutritional status than a child from a poor household which has increased over time from 1992-93 to 2005-06. However maximum household level heterogeneity in socioeconomic impact on stunting is visible in MPHI states even after controlling child, mother and household level characteristics.

Table 13: Percentage variance contribution of community and household level in total variance in four models in 1992-93, 1998-99 and 2005-06 in India and HPHI, HPMI, HPLI and MPHI states in 2005-06

% contribution of two levels in total variance		*Model Null*	*Model Kid*	*Model Mother*	*Model Household*
NFHS I	PSU	0.65	0.50	0.48	0.48
	Household	0.35	0.50	0.52	0.52
NFHS II	PSU	0.11	0.07	0.07	0.08
	Household	0.89	0.93	0.93	0.92
NFHS III	PSU	0.31	0.20	0.17	0.18
	Household	0.69	0.80	0.83	0.82
HPHI	PSU	0.39	0.30	0.35	0.34
	Household	0.61	0.70	0.65	0.66
HPMI	PSU	0.25	0.22	0.18	0.18
	Household	0.75	0.78	0.82	0.82
HPLI	PSU	0.39	0.2	0.19	0.21
	Household	0.61	0.8	0.81	0.79
MPHI	PSU	0.10	0.07	0.06	0.06
	Household	0.90	0.93	0.94	0.94

CONTRIBUTION OF DIFFERENT FACTORS IN INEQUITY IN NUTRITIONAL STATUS

Table 14 shows pattern of contribution of different factors in inequity in stunting among children under the age of three in fifteen major states of India. In all the time points, major contributing factors are socioeconomic status, mother's education and mother's contact to health service delivery. During the period of one and half decade, contribution of socioeconomic status has been increased by two percentage points. However, from first to second time point direct contribution of SLI has fallen by fifteen percentage points and the same of mother's education and access to healthcare has been increased by two and one percentage points respectively. But from second to third time point, SLI direct contribution has been increased by seventeen percentage points. Whereas, the same of mother's knowledge has been decreased by eleven percentage points and contribution of contact to health service remain the same.

Since, decomposition results at the all India level are not showing any clear pattern, I perform the decomposition for fifteen major states for three time points (Table 15). It is evident that for nine states shown under green area, the contribution of socioeconomic status has declined. For three states, there is marginal increase (shown under yellow area). In Rajasthan, West Bengal and Madhya Pradesh there is substantial increase in the contribution of socioeconomic status in inequity in nutritional achievement of children (shown under orange area). Therefore, I can infer that statewise heterogeneous pattern of contribution of socioeconomic status is responsible for showing no particular pattern at country level. Since, increasing pattern is visible in smaller number of states, therefore that influence gets cancelled out by decreasing pattern visible in higher number of states.

Discussion

This chapter tries to see the pattern of change in socioeconomic gradient in stunting in India in one and half decade as it is not

Table 14: Concentration Index (CI) decomposition results for three time points showing pattern of contribution of different factors in inequity in nutritional status over three time points

	1992-93				*1998-99*				*2005-06*			
Factor	***Elasticity***	***CI***	***Contribution***	***% Contribution***	***Elasticity***	***CI***	***Contribution***	***% Contribution***	***Elasticity***	***CI***	***Contribution***	***% Contribution***
Age	0.614	0.003	0.002	–0.030	0.655	0.004	0.003	–0.038	–	–	–	–
Sex	–0.096	–0.002	0.000	–0.003	–0.025	–0.003	0.000	–0.001	–	–	–	–
Birth order	0.039	–0.032	–0.001	0.021	0.049	–0.040	–0.002	0.029	0.055	–0.055	–0.003	0.033
Size of the child at birth	0.197	–0.004	–0.001	0.014	0.226	–0.009	–0.002	0.029	0.149	–0.013	–0.002	0.021
Exclusive breast-feeding	0.000	–0.148	0.000	–0.001	–0.004	–0.117	0.001	–0.008	–0.007	–0.114	0.000	-0.009
Complementary feeding	0.016	–0.025	0.000	0.007	0.022	0.012	0.000	–0.004	–0.081	0.013	–0.001	0.012
SLI	–0.115	0.235	–0.027	0.472	–0.103	0.204	–0.021	0.317	–0.196	0.227	–0.044	0.488
Mother's education	–0.058	0.356	–0.021	0.365	–0.081	0.316	–0.026	0.386	–0.091	0.280	–0.025	0.279
Mother's occupational status	0.003	–0.161	0.000	0.008	–0.001	–0.172	0.000	–0.004	0.015	–0.127	–0.002	0.021
Place of delivery	–0.134	0.056	–0.008	0.132	–0.155	0.057	–0.009	0.135	–0.154	0.081	–0.013	0.137
Religion	0.008	–0.004	0.000	0.001	–0.002	–0.016	0.000	0.000	–0.017	–0.013	0.000	–0.002
Caste	–0.001	–0.183	0.000	–0.002	0.031	–0.105	–0.003	0.050	0.048	–0.087	–0.004	0.046
Impact of location	0.164	–0.033	–0.005	0.094	0.224	–0.041	–0.009	0.138	–0.003	–0.066	0.000	–0.002
Community fixed effect	–	–	0.003	–0.047	–	–	0.002	–0.028	–	–	0.000	0.002
Residual	–	–	0.002	–	–	–	0.000	–	–	–	0.000	–

Table 15: Concentration Index (CI) decomposition results for three time points showing pattern of contribution of socioeconomic status in inequity in nutritional status over three time points

	NFHS1	*NFHS2*	*NFHS3*
Assam	0.41	–0.42	–0.44
Bihar	0.46	0.31	–0.04
Gujarat	0.88	0.41	0.78
Haryana	0.57	0.33	0.51
Karnataka	0.74	–0.02	0.37
Orissa	0.53	0.63	0.45
Punjab	0.76	–0.04	0.45
Tamil Nadu	0.70	0.82	0.43
Uttar Pradesh	–0.31	0.32	0.31
Andhra Pradesh	0.61	0.22	0.65
Kerala	0.82	0.42	0.86
Maharashtra	0.40	0.67	0.46
Madhya Pradesh	0.40	0.45	0.51
Rajasthan	–0.85	0.3	0.57
West Bengal	0.52	0.21	0.68

Source: Three NFHS rounds

explored yet. It also explores the determinants of stunting in major states by clubbing them into groups based on certain criteria. The results of the chapter show significant increase in inequity in nutritional status among children under the age of three in fifteen major Indian states in three time points. Decline in stunting prevalence is higher in richer families implying widening of inequity among poor and rich. Seeing the scenario it is evident that burden of absolute inequity is higher in HPHI and HPLI state groups. Variance contributions reconfirm existence of socioeconomic gradient. It shows a non-linear pattern of change in strength of the gradient with steep increase in strength in first five years and then a little arrest in next five years though the degree of strength is much higher in 2005-06 compared to 1992-93. Household level inequity is highest in MPHI states compared to other state groups.

Inequity related to child's age, sex, number of children in a family, size of the child at birth as a proxy of birth weight, introduction of complementary feeding in timely manner, and mother's care giving knowledge, attitudes and practices are common in major states as determinants of stunting. Inequity in relation to mother's employment status is one significant influencing factor in HPMI (Gujarat, Andhra Pradesh, Karnataka, and Tamil Nadu) and HPLI states (Uttar Pradesh, Madhya Pradesh, Rajasthan, Bihar and Assam). In the above major states and MPHI states (Punjab, Haryana, West Bengal, Maharashtra, and Kerala) contact with health service is significantly influencing the nutritional status of children. One study confirms that if mother's contact with health service is better, then there is probability of reduction in stunting in HPMI and HPLI states (Brennan *et al.*, 2004). These results will be explained in detail in the light of different earlier works on developing countries in general and India in particular.

Incorporation of child's characteristics, mother's characteristics reduces the impact of socioeconomic status. Thus SLI works through these factors. Therefore where the reason is age or mother's education, basically, illiterate mothers belong to poor families and thus it is SLI which is the main influencing factor as found in previous work (Kanjilal *et al.*, 2010). As for example, in Orissa mother's education is a strong confounder so health seeking is not visibly significant here (Kesterton *et al.*, 2010). In Orissa near about 60 percent children are delivered at home according to NFHS III (IIPS, 2007). Thus mothers' less utilization of health facility may be one cause of poor childcare as evident in other developing countries (Sakisaka *et al.,* 2010). Another point is weaning period children are more undernourished significantly in 2005-06. Complementary feeding practice is significant in 2005-06 in HPMI and HPLI states and controlling it reduces the direct marginal impact of socioeconomic status as poor children of weaning period do late and/or improper start of semi-solid or solid food (Padmadas *et al.,* 2002; Anoop *et al.,* 2004). Thus socioeconomic factor is the main player here which works through child's age, feeding practice and mother's education which is also in line with other previous studies (Hong *et al.,* 2006; Svedberg, 2008).

In HPLI and MPHI states, household's social status is a significant influencing factor. In HPLI states, socioeconomic gradient is working through the pathway of social heterogeneity. But in MPHI states, social inequity is confounding the impact of economic inequity. In HPLI states most of the children are undernourished. According to Census (2011), population composition of these states show that significant percentage of rural population constitutes backward caste population. In MPHI states not only poor population of general community is stunted but significant percentage of backward caste child population living in different pockets are also undernourished.

In HPHI state Orissa, though it is evident from earlier study (Sharma *et al.*, 2009) that there is a good reduction in under-nutrition percentage, fall in infant mortality rate, improvement in childcare and feeding practice indicators (*e.g.*, breastfeeding and complementary feeding); the under-nutrition prevalence is still high with high socioeconomic inequity. It is visible from NFHS III (IIPS, 2007) that poor social status along with living under dismal poverty; infant and child mortality, stunting –all are highest among scheduled tribe, scheduled caste, other backward caste, children living in poor environment and among rural children. Traditions, cultures and practices vary across caste/ethnic groups, and some of these variations have a bearing on acceptability of maternal and child healthcare (Caldwell, 1993; ICMR, 2003; Ghosh, 2012). All this diversity poses a challenge for service providers in the state (Peters *et al.*, 2008). Irrespective of efforts and strategies to address determinants there remains a huge gap and the multi-factorial causes of under-nutrition can only be partially ameliorated by any one scheme or department (Sharma *et al.*, 2009).

Major findings related to MPHI states are, household level heterogeneity in relation to socioeconomic gradient of stunting is highest even after controlling for several child, mother and household factor related inequity. Economic and social status of household are strong influencing factors contributing to inequity as poor and tribal people seek less care from qualified provider governed by their traditional culture, resource scarce environment and livelihood insecurity visible among tribal population of Maharashtra (Sonowal, 2010). Another point deserves mention that MPHI states show that urban children are more undernourished than rural children in the model which may be the confounding effect of unobserved factors so it requires further research taking at least the state with highest rural urban disparity in prevalence and/or inequity.

Thus it is clear that observing the importance of access barriers to healthcare seeking related health interventions have improved mother's knowledge and health seeking but condition of poor remain worse with respect to basic amenities including health. If I look back to history of health interventions to reduce inequity in health - propelled by several structural inequities after globalization and structural adjustment programmes, such interventions remain insufficient and less successful (Gopalan *et al.,* 2011). For success, resource allocation need to be optimal *i.e.,* will cater to various determinants of health (water, sanitation, housing, livelihood) other than healthcare (ibid.). But from this study it is clear that policies on health equity, which follows a holistic approach to achieve inclusive growth (growth along with socioeconomic development) and expected to accelerate the pace to achieve Millennium Development Goals is not either properly designed or implemented as also reviewed in other previous study (ibid.).

Therefore whether policy process in India has followed equity approach to bring integrated health sector reform following Alma Ata Declaration and United Nations Millennium declaration is needed to be explored more. To investigate the same, several previous research works and policy documents studied the policy determinatives, whole health policy process – from agenda setting, policy development, implementation, evaluation, and policy outcome (Walt *et al.,* 2008, Gopalan *et al.,* 2011). The literatures concentrated on looking at how far social determinants of health are included comprehensively, whether participatory policy processes are included or not, if included then to what extent, how far evidences on health inequity among vulnerable groups are generated and used, how much the policy was oriented to bring equitable, timely, acceptable and affordable healthcare services for vulnerable groups (ibid.). But such analysis is required at more micro level.

It is clear from my study that vulnerable population in terms of social status (backward caste), economic status (poor children) and location of residence (rural area) are not targeted properly using health equity approach as found in few earlier works on India and other developing country context (Mahal *et al.*, 2001; Steinhardt *et al.,* 2009; Sinha *et al.,* 2009; Das *et al.,* 2010). Though under such approach, health seeking behaviour and awareness about childcare is improved to some extent, still the poor children are in worse situation due to several poverty syndrome factors – poor living environment, less health seeking due to lack of knowledge, traditional culture and higher opportunity cost like other developing countries as well as results from studies on India (Smith and Haddad, 1999; Svedberg, 2000; 2006; 2008; Larrea and Freire, 2002; Zere and McIntyre, 2003; Deolalikar, 2004; Navaneetham and Jose, 2005; Hong and Mishra, 2006; Hong *et al.*, 2006; Fotso, 2006; Pongou *et al.*, 2006; Poel *et al.*, 2008; Taguri *et al.*, 2008; Kanjilal *et al.*, 2010). Thus poverty syndrome is a major hindrance to achieve health equity through improvement of vulnerable population (Peters *et al.*, 2008; Steinhardt *et al.*, 2009). Therefore, the fundamental remedy is optimal allocation of physical, financial, and managerial resources to ensure universal coverage with effective service delivery, strong monitoring and periodic evaluation through effective governance (Braveman, 2006; Gopalan *et al.*, 2011).

One intervention can be use of health information technology to improve the monitoring of the Government at all levels – from grassroot frontline workers to central ministry. This can improve the service delivery through increasing the efficacy of governance with respect to nutrition service delivery system in India. From

1975, India Government runs one big programme – Integrated Child Development Service – to improve the nutritional status of children in India but it is not successful to eradicate inequity in nutritional status even it is pro-poor and pro-marginalised. One major reason is, data collected at ground level by anganwadi workers in ICDS centers do not reach at central level where policy decisions are taken care of. Because at each level of hierarchy, data is aggregated for the next level official and gradually the individual level information remain hidden in aggregated averages. If through the help of information technology, the ground level individual specific data can be entered into a system which will be visible up to central level then it will be easy for policy makers to build strategies depending on the ground level situation. They can easily decide on which pocket needs special attention with what specific intervention like which state pocket needs more awareness generating counseling sessions, which one needs more supply of food and/or medicines, more human resource etc. Therefore through e-governance method the inclusive growth can be accelerated.

5

Contextually Vulnerable Area: The Sundarbans Delta Case Study

BACKGROUND

As per previous chapter analyses, medium prevalent high inequity states are more vulnerable in terms of household level inequity in nutritional achievement among children. As one MPHI state, West Bengal shows higher contribution of SES gradient in inequity with higher increase in contribution, and also higher rural urban disparity in inequity in nutritional achievement (Mukherjee, 2015). Therefore, if we explore vulnerable rural pockets and the urban areas, we could be able to assess the prime and distal factors behind, their complex pathways and therefore could suggest effective policies. The Sundarbans delta region is one such rural vulnerable pocket which is the focus of my work here[1].

THE CONTEXT

'The Sundarbans', a density of Sundari trees, is known as 'Sodorbon' (in local terminology). The area is not uni-characteristic; it is a conglomeration of multidimensional diversities. It is a land of

[1] Funded by SRTT fellowship, ISEC, Bangalore

adverse features as well. Such poetic co-habitat of 'beauty and the beast' is rare across the globe. Fishermen risk their lives inside the unknown world of sea everyday, woodcutters roll deep into the dense forest to bring wood for making their lives. The habitats collect their inspiration of life, happiness and joy from the emotion that evolves from the unavoidable brutal reality of the geography. The cult and culture of the Sundarbans is reflected in the epistle of international and national tourists since ages. Some of them are – Romila Thapar, Bipan Chanda, Ramsharan Sharma, Goutam Bhadra and similar others. Population of the Sundarbans is of mixed nature. People from various regions of West Bengal migrated to the Sundarbans to earn their livelihood, especially who were landless and poverty-stricken. Exploitation, tyranny, poverty and ignorance generated food insecurity and famine.

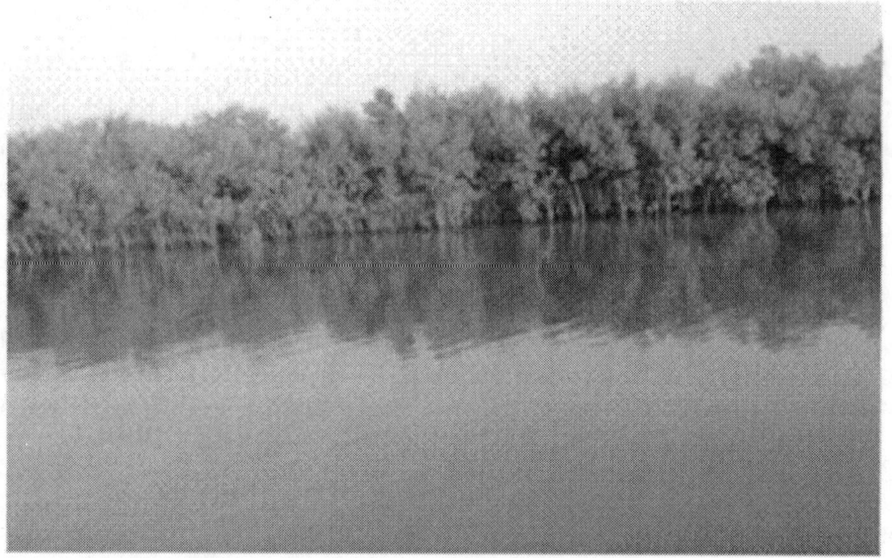

Two-third of the Sundarbans is in Bangladesh and the rest is in West Bengal. In the Indian part, the total area of the Sundarbans is 9630 sq km, of which 5700 sq km area is land and 4264 sq km area is covered with mangroves. The archipelago consists of 104 islands of which 54 islands have human existence and the non-deltaic part is connected to the mainland. A number of rivers and estuaries have intersected the area from north to south and narrow tidal creeks from east to west (IIHMR, 2010). Around 29-30 violent cyclones exploded in the region between 1960 and 2010.

The Sundarbans National Park is a famous Tiger Reserve and a unique biosphere reserve. In 1973, 'Sundarban Development Board' was founded to attend the misery, illiteracy and poor health of the inhabitants, and also for repairing the embankments and transport system. Although quite a few have been implemented, there are still a wide gap between targets and achievements.

Health in the Sundarbans

The geo-volatility of the Sundarbans makes it special not only with respect to livelihood and survival of its people but also in terms of people's health status. A typical resident of the Sundarbans carries an extra load of ill-health and health risks compared to others living within the same district. As it has been found, the children are the worst sufferers; most of them are chronically malnourished and, hence, perennially suffer from disproportionately higher burden of respiratory and gastro-enteric troubles (IIIHMR, 2010). In brief, with about 4 million people currently estimated to live in the region, this neglected population has become a major reservoir for a wide spectrum of health conditions that are not always well recognized by the existing formal health sector (ibid.).

In this backdrop, my study is a little initiative to depict the under-nutrition and morbidity pattern through a pilot study and I explored its determinants to help the policymakers in designing future enterprise.

Hypothesis

The contextual uncertainties[2] coupled with demographic characteristics, livelihood insecurity, chronic poverty, culture,

[2] Geographical, climatic, socioeconomic vulnerabilities

collectiveness and supply side environment[3] are associated with the under-nutrition levels and morbidity in the Sundarbans, West Bengal.

Research Objectives

- General objective - Explore the contextual determinants of under-nutrition and related morbidities among children under the age of five in the two villages of two GPs in the Patharprtima block of the Sundarbans based on the WHO growth standard
- To reach the general objective the specific objectives are -
    - Assess the degrees of contextual uncertainties influencing the prevalence of under-nutrition and morbidity among children under the age of five
    - Assess whether and by what degree the impact of uncertainties differs by climatic shock, geographical adversities, livelihood insecurities, culture and collectiveness as well as supply side environment over socioeconomic status (SES), caste, demography of children as well as mother related factors

METHODOLOGY

The Study Area

The area for the research study was selected based on geographic location (deltaic or non-deltaic[4]), percentage of poor and marginalized population, availability of transport and village infrastructure as it was hypothesized that delta region suffers more due to climatic shock induced physical inaccessibility and

---

[3] It denotes the Integrated Child Development Service (ICDS) service delivery system

[4] Deltaic – Area surrounded by water (river/ sea/ creeks), Non-deltaic – Area which is at least connected to mainland at one side

vulnerability to poverty compared to non-deltaic region (Figure 5:1). The Patharpratima block of the Sundarbans region under the administrative jurisdiction of South 24 Parganas district of West Bengal consists of 162300 male population, 154618 female population, among which 24 percent is Scheduled Caste and 1 percent is Scheduled Tribe population (Projected population from Census, 2001). The selected Gram Panchayets from the block - G Plot is the deltaic GP and Ramganga is the non-deltaic GP. In the selected village of Rajrajeswarpur of Ramganga GP 52 percent and in the another selected village Krishnadaspur of G Plot GP 60 percent population belongs to SC and ST category as per projected population calculated on 2001 Census figure.

Village Details

Krishnadaspur- This village is located in deltaic gram panchayet G-Plot (the white spot on the northern part of the GP). According to key informant interview, the village is around 3.5 km away from GP Headquarter and people have to spend approximately one hour to reach the block town from the centre of the village. Within 4km of distance, they can access Sub Centre, Primary School, ICDS Centre, RMP Clinic and traditional healers (*e.g.* Ojha, Gunin). Nearest Primary Health Centre is within 7-8 km distance. Madhabnagar BPHC is located 20-25 km far away. One NGO provides social services related to health, education and livelihood in the village. Nearest Bus Stand is in Ramganga; villagers have to travel for more than two hours to reach there.

We also asked about condition of physical infrastructure of the village. Maximum roads are either muddy with suboptimal condition or concrete/brick bound roads are in poor condition due to lack of maintenance. Embankments on rivers are mostly temporary in nature and concrete embankments scarcely exist. There is no temporary or concrete bridge on the river. Drinking water supply is not well developed. The drinking water source is hand pump with platform instead of piped water supply or deep tube well. Drinking water collection from open or closed well was

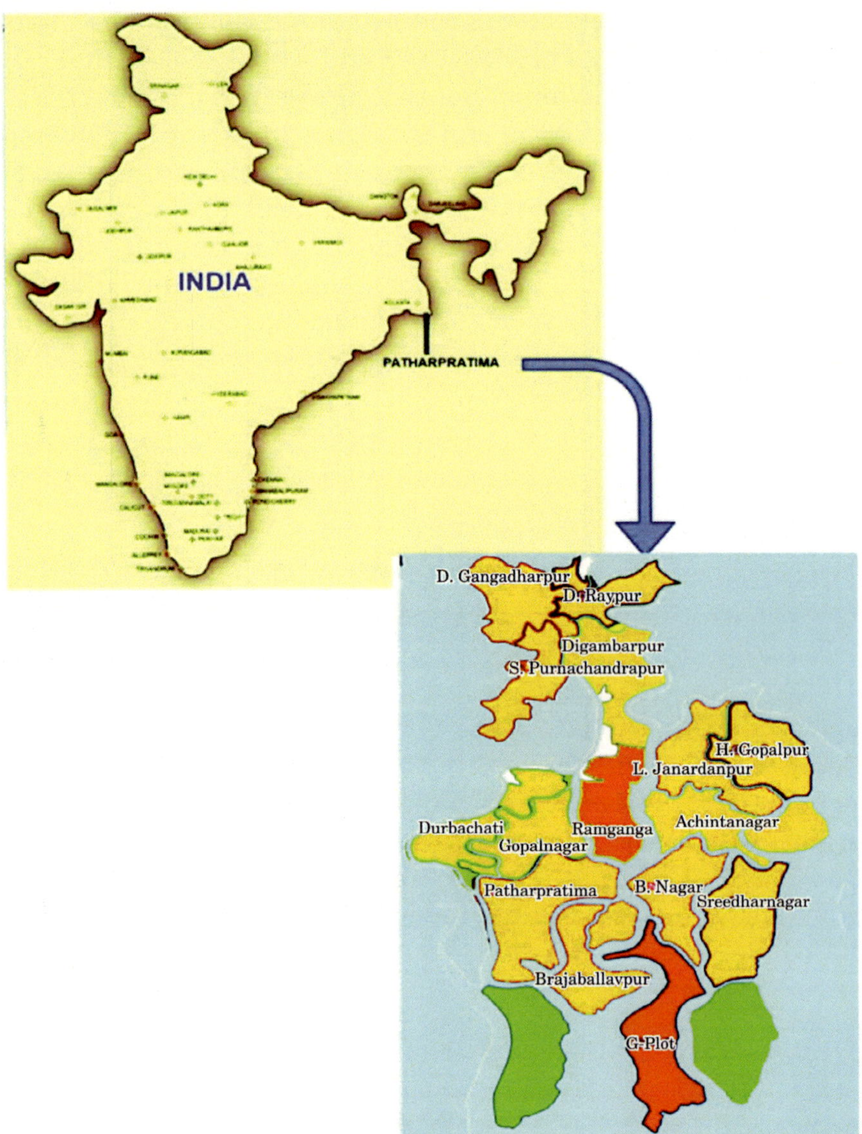

Figure 5.1: The Study Area Taken from IIHMR Report on Patharpratima 2011 and The Sundarbans Report, ISEC 2014.

never practiced in the village. Inhabitants mostly defecate in pucca or kutcha open latrine and toilets with or without safety tank which are in partially good condition. Electric lines for domestic consumption for common people, for commercial consumption for business and telecommunication services are never existed. Tall concrete building used as shelter during floods/water logging is in suboptimal condition. According to Focused Group Discussion following key informant's report, climatic shock worsens the infrastructure and assets to a great extent. Land fertility overall as well as near coastal area is affected by increased salinity and little production takes place. Drinking water source gets contaminated and water becomes scarce during and after climatic shock.

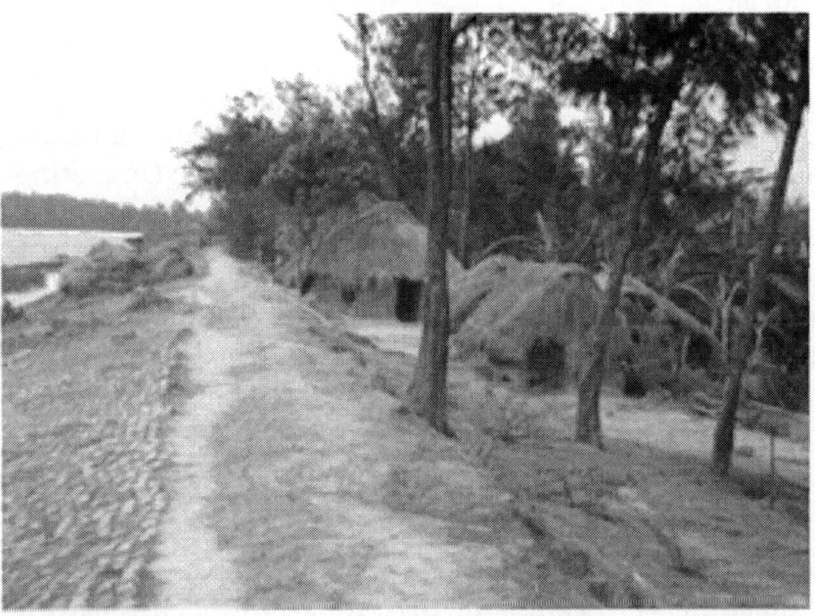

Regarding existence of shops or market place, religious centre and community centre, he reported that though a market exists it is non-functional, religious centres exist and functional but community centre does not exist. According to him, market is non-functional because demand for food or other materials is limited as inhabitants purchase food once or twice in a week and purchase other commodities like clothes and other goods occasionally. Most of the inhabitants do not purchase due to lack of purchasing power.

In relation to availability of public transport he said that van/ rickshaw, motor van, boat or ferry serves infrequently, auto-rickshaw, bus or train never exist. Walking or running any vehicle during rainy season or during and after flood or cyclone becomes extremely difficult. Concerning experience of the community about health and nutrition service delivery during last 12 months preceding the survey, it is evident that frequent or unjustified absence of doctors and other staffs, irregular home visits by frontline workers, avoid of visit in hard to reach areas, poor service during emergency, and drug shortage in hospital are common scenario.

Inside the village community, religious centres, Self Help Groups, Political party clubs exist. Majority of the people living within the community take benefit from these organizations or some only have connections. Participating in SHG meetings they become aware about their rights and started earning through different livelihood approaches. Political groups or clubs mainly help during emergency situation. Connections with NGOs/CBOs help to build new contacts and help during emergency serving food and healthcare. Religious centres are mainly community specific whereas SHG members and political clubs work across communities.

Rajrajeswarpur- It is located in non-deltaic Gram Panchayet Ramganga (the white dot on the north-eastern part of the GP). Distance of GP headquarter is 4 km from the centre of the village. By machine van, centre of the village to block town takes 20 minutes. Within 1 km of distance they can access primary and secondary schools, four ICDS centres, bus stand, ferry ghat, and five to six traditional healers. Within two kilometres of distance they can access Sub Centre and RMP clinic. Panchayet office is located at the distance of 5-7 km and Block Primary Health Centre is 10 km away from there. Two NGOs Sundarban Social Development Centre and Indranarayanpur Nazrul Smriti Sangha provide social services related to health, water and sanitation, education, and livelihood.

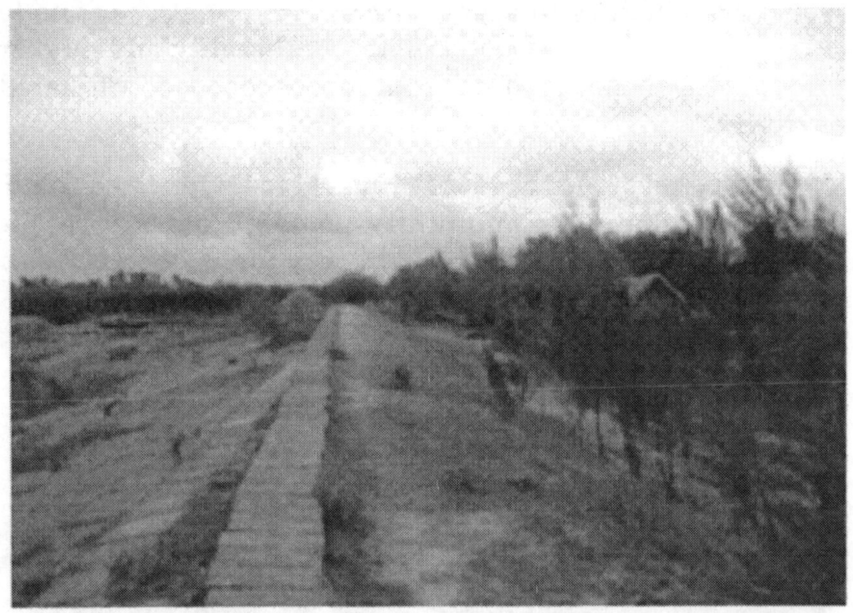

Regarding physical infrastructure, the key informant reported that muddy roads scarcely exist and most of the roads are either brick bound or concrete but frequent climatic shock damages the roads and poor maintenance due to lack of initiative is evident. There is no temporary embankment; concrete embankment exists with sub-optimal condition due to damage after cyclones along with lack of initiatives for maintaining it properly. Bridge (temporary/ concrete), piped water, deep tube well never existed due to lack of initiatives. Hand pump is the main source of drinking water which is also not maintained properly. Well never existed. Toilet with safety tank does not exist and without safety tank scarcely exist. Eighty percent villagers use pucca open latrine, 2 percent uses kutcha open latrine and rest uses bush for defecation. Electricity has come last year for domestic consumption but they experience frequent power cut for 5-6 hours in every 3-4 days a week. Electricity for commercial consumption and telecommunication exists. No concrete building is there to provide shelter except the high school building during cyclones and floods. Climatic shock worsens land fertility to a great extent and quality of the land near coastal area gets affected more. Availability and quality of water used for drinking or other purposes gets contaminated to some extent.

Regarding existence of shops or markets he reported that it is currently developing. Community people celebrate religious festivals once in a year and they are very much devoted to their religion. No community centre is present.

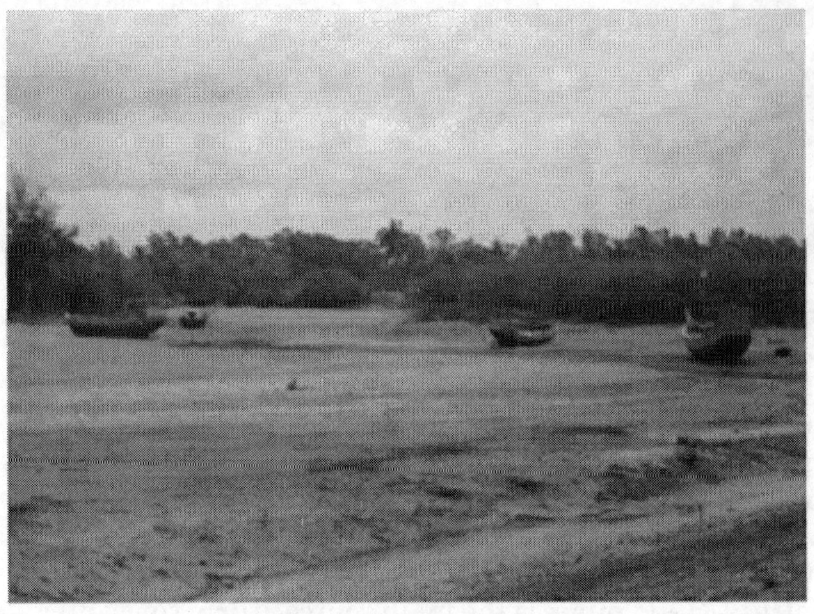

Regarding quality of transport, he reported that van and motor van, boat or ferry are available all the time. Auto-rickshaw is not available. Bus is available. There is no train service. He also said that road accessibility during rainy season does not become so difficult since road condition has improved for last one year. He also reported about the prevailing community perceptions regarding health and nutrition service delivery during the last 12 months preceding the survey. Most of the villagers experience frequent and unjustified absence of doctors, home visit of anganwadi workers are done, no or limited service is available during emergency, drug shortage in hospital, food shortage in AWC and crowding of hospitals are very common.

The community consists of religious centres, Self Help Groups, Political Party Clubs and NGOs, CBOs. They mostly gather for recreation or building new contacts or relationships. They generally get benefited from SHG members in developing awareness regarding livelihood and childcare.

DATA COLLECTION

To test the study hypothesis, I have collected information on village infrastructure, community perception about health and nutrition service delivery and community characteristics at village level. It is collected through one structured questionnaire and in-depth interview of one village leader in each village. The household level information is collected using a structured questionnaire covering socioeconomic and demographic profile of household members; impact of climatic shock on household assets, physical infrastructure, and healthcare access; mother and child's health seeking behaviour, mother's perception about child health and nutrition status, awareness, childcare and feeding practice, effectiveness of anganwadi services *e.g.*, anganwadi worker's (AWW) visits, frequency of visits, type of suggestions given by them to the mothers and caregivers, frequency of receiving supplementary food, whether child eat the food, food is shared or not. Also information is collected on what is the amount of healthcare expenditure to cover treatment of their children, whether households' perception about economic status fall differs from actual economic status fall. Their perception about food insecurity and increase in healthcare spending during climatic shock has also been collected to find whether any association between climatic shock and under-nutrition exists which works through the pathway of their perception in the study area. In addition to this, I have done one Focused Group Discussion of mothers/caregivers, one Focused Group Discussion of earning members, and one in-depth interview of frontline worker in each village.

METHODS

The data collection is done following stratified random sampling technique where the block is stratified into two strata - deltaic region and non-deltaic region. From deltaic region, I have selected G-Plot gram panchayet which is one of the most vulnerable GPs in the Patharpratima block with respect to geographic location - connection with block headquarter, availability and accessibility of transport. The GP is very much threaten by impacts of climate change induced climatic shock which caused disappearing of one village Gobardhanpur inside the sea 10-12 years ago. "The southern part of Sitarampur has disappeared, while the northern part is slowly getting swallowed up as the land gets eroded by the onslaught of the sea." – The Hindu, Feb 24, 2008. Among 9 villages in G Plot GP, I selected Krishnadaspur based on the criterion of higher marginalized population. Comparatively, Ramganga GP is located in the main land and straight connected to the other developed blocks of the district. So it is comparatively well off with respect to access dimension. Among 10 villages of this GP, I selected Rajrajeswarpur village based on the same criterion.

SAMPLING

Observing that deltaic population lives with much geographical adversities compared to non-deltaic population, delta and non-delta stratification under stratified random sampling is justified. After selection of Krishnadaspur and Rajrajeswarpur villages based on the Schedule Caste and Schedule Tribe population and degree of impact of climatic events, I estimated the sample size to test my hypothesis. I did the household survey in that vulnerable block (identified according to service delivery space and accessibility index in FHS 2010) – Patharpratima Block in the

Sundarbans during 2013. The household survey was a cross-section study covering the villages from the deltaic Gram Panchayat and the non-deltaic Gram Panchayat. Following method was used to collect the data. Therefore the block is divided into two strata based on the geographic location, climatic shock proneness of GPs. The two strata are 1) Deltaic and 2) non-deltaic. The sample size calculation is based on three factors (i) the child (0-6 years) population in the block (ii) the desired level of confidence and (iii) the acceptable margin of error. Hence the required sample size will be calculated using formula,

$$n= \{t^2 \times p(1-p) \times d\}/m^2$$

where,

n = required sample size

t = confidence level at 95% (standard value of 1.96)

p = Prevalence of stunting (0-5 years) (Based on FHS 2010 survey)

m = margin of error at 5% (standard value of 0.05)

d= design effect (taken as 2- the default value).

Thus n=767.

In total 840 children (0-5 years) is the sample size after doing 10% oversampling. From two villages in two GPs I collected information of 336 households (40 percent of total sample – 168 households from each village). I collected information for total 338 youngest living children from 338 households.

Analytical Method

First, qualitative data was analysed manually. Quantitative data was edited in the field and cleaned. Data analysis was done using STATA 11 package to know the sample characteristics, background characteristics of the respondents, cross-tabulation results of outcome variables by background characteristics, regression analyses to find the significant influencing factors with confounders. It explored whether there exists any delta-non delta variation in health outcome and nutritional outcome with respect to contextual uncertainties and supply side environment. I used conventional anthropometric measure height for age indicator (stunting[5]) according to WHO reference population. Analysis is done to see whether contribution to the heterogeneous health and nutrition outcome is attributed to household level more than the village level and whether extreme climatic events aggravate health shock and increase the likelihood of under-nutrition and whether related coping strategies influence the childcare and feeding and thereby increase the complexities through the pathway of mother's perception.

To make the analysis transparent, I prepared some indices. One is perceived poverty index prepared from variables where I asked questions – "In terms of the ability to meet the annual food consumption needs of the household, where would you place your household?", "Have all of your household members including you had full two square meals/sufficient meals every day for the last seven days?", "How do you compare your household income- in the last one year in relation to your Household expenditure?". Based on the options, I ran principal component factor analysis which showed scale reliability coefficient is 0.65 and loaded most of the variables in 'factor one' and based on this factor score I created perceived poverty index where three categories are most poor, medium poor and least poor.

To rank and categorise the mothers according to their health seeking behaviour, I created another index representing their contact to health facility. The variables represent the number of ante-natal care taken and place of delivery of the youngest child. The alpha value obtained before factor analysis was 0.59 and three

[5] Since stunting represents chronic nutritional deprivation, impact of contextual uncertainties including chronic poverty can be better captured using this indicator.

categories of the index shows poor contact, medium contact and good contact.

To estimate whether the under-nutrition is more or less likely associated with contextual vulnerabilities, I created Climate Impact Index (CII), Livelihood Insecurity Index (LII), Physical Inaccessibility Index (PII), and Treatment Seeking Vulnerability Index (TSVI). CII was created using variables measuring – impact of cyclone and flood on household's house and productive assets categorized as per (a) perceived poverty trend with categories-less vulnerable with devastation, vulnerable with partial damage, more vulnerable and devastated; (b) perception about change in healthcare expenditure during climatic shock with categories- not at all, sometimes in devastated family, more often in devastated family, to a great extent in devastated family and experience with no or partial damage, (c) actual economic status fall due to healthcare spending with categories severe fall with devastation, moderate fall with devastation, some fall with devastation, status fall experience with no or partial damage. Two other variables used are household's perception about degree of impact on housing and drinking water supply. The alpha value shows that scale reliability coefficient is 0.63. Score of factor 1 is categorized into three- most vulnerable, medium vulnerable and least vulnerable.

LII was created using the variables measuring the degree of impact (quantifying the quality indicators) of climatic shock on livestock, land and crop, on degree of barrenness of land, difficulty in fishing, livestock rearing, wood cutting or honey collection. The value of scale reliability coefficient is 0.67. The three categories of first factor score are most vulnerable, medium vulnerable and least vulnerable.

PII is created using variables measuring the degree of impact of climatic shock on village road, transport facility on land and water, access to Government health facility/hospital, caused no transport facility or damaged road. Other variables used are inability to access facility due to distance, the mode of transport used to access health facility – walking, by boat, launch, van, small trekker (magic van in local terminology), and bus. The value of scale reliability coefficient is 0.82. The three categories of first factor score are most difficult to access, medium difficulty to access, least difficulty to access.

TSVI is created using variables quantifying the perception of households regarding availability of medicine and other goods and patient loads in Government hospitals, variation in treatment cost in RMP clinic during climatic shock, whether health condition of child deteriorates after treatment seeking near RMPs, keeping children treated under home remedy is better if RMP treatment is risky and increases frequency of illness, whether treating under qualified provider is better; and the variables - preference pattern about child's delivery when experiencing obstetric complications during climatic shock with options home delivery with dai or RMP or institution, behaviour of RMPs during treatment seeking. The scale reliability coefficient is 0.68. The factor 1 score is categorized into most vulnerable, medium vulnerable and least vulnerable.

6

Socioeconomic, Demographic Profile of the Inhabitants and Prevalence of Gastroenteric Morbidity and Stunting in the Study Area

This chapter deals with the background profile of the inhabitants in the two villages. Below table (Table# 16) presents the socioeconomic profile of inhabitants in the study area. Inhabitants of the two study villages in the two GPs of the Patharpratima block live below the poverty line according to the World Bank definition of poverty line. I also have estimated their perception about their own economic status. According to Perceived Poverty Index which shows that the village of the deltaic GP has marginally higher population of most poor (35 percent in Krishnadaspur and 34.6 percent in Rajrajeswarpur). Based on trajectory of poverty perception, smooth pattern of persisting chronic poverty is highly evident within Krishnadaspur compared to Rajrajeswarpur. Whereas oscillated deepening of chronic poverty is higher in the village of non-deltaic GP (52 percent). But gradual deepening is higher among inhabitants of deltaic GP (26 percent). Two out of three families in deltaic village and half of the families in non-deltaic village spends 2000 to 3000 rupees for covering monthly consumption. Higher level of monthly consumption expenditure is visible among least poor community in non-deltaic village.

Table# 16: Socioeconomic profile of the inhabitants in the two villages in the two GPs of the Patharpratima block

	G - Plot		*Ramganga*		*Total*	
	Krishnadaspur		*Rajrajeswarpur*			
	N	%	*N*	%	*N*	%
Perceived Poverty						
Most Poor	55	35.0	55	34.6	110	34.8
Medium	55	35.0	56	35.2	111	35.1
Least Poor	47	29.9	48	30.2	95	30.1
Trajectory of Poverty perception						
Smooth pattern of chronic poverty	21	13.1	7	4.2	28	8.6
Smooth movement towards poverty line	7	4.4	7	4.2	14	4.3
Oscillated deepening of chronic poverty (declining saw-tooth)	50	31.3	87	52.1	137	41.9
Smooth abrupt deepening of chronic poverty	29	18.1	20	12.0	49	15.0
Gradual deepening of chronic poverty	42	26.3	24	14.4	66	20.2
Oscillated movemen't towards poverty line (improving saw-tooth)	11	6.9	22	13.2	33	10.1
Monthly consumption expenditure						
Rs. 500-2000	19	11.5	26	15.6	45	13.5
Rs. 2001-3000	103	62.1	84	50.3	187	56.2
Rs. 3000 & above	44	26.5	57	34.1	101	30.3
Family Type						
Nuclear	135	80.8	111	66.5	246	73.7
Joint	32	19.2	56	33.5	88	26.4
House Type						
Kutcha	153	91.6	147	88.0	300	89.8
Semi-Pucca	6	3.59	15	9.0	21	6.3
Pucca	8	4.79	5	3.0	13	3.9
Number of rooms						
One	101	60.5	57	34.1	158	47.3
Two	60	35.9	86	51.5	146	43.7
More than two	6	3.6	24	14.4	30	9.0
Type of Cooking Fuel						
Wood	3	1.8	6	3.6	9	2.7

Table# 16: (*Contd...*)

Table# 16: *(Contd...)*

	G - Plot		*Ramganga*		*Total*	
	Krishnadaspur		*Rajrajeswarpur*			
	N	*%*	*N*	*%*	*N*	*%*
Crop residues	161	95.8	139	82.7	300	89.3
Cow dung cakes	4	2.4	22	13.1	26	7.7
Liquid petroleum gas	0	0.0	1	0.6	1	0.3
Drinking Water Source						
Open well	1	0.6	0	0	1	0.3
Tube well	166	98.8	168	100	334	99.4
Tap/deep	1	0.6	0	0	1	0.3
Type of latrine						
Sanitary latrine –Yes	100	59.2	117	69.2	217	64.2
No	69	40.8	52	30.8	121	35.8
Electricity						
Yes	77	45.6	115	68.1	192	56.8
No	92	54.4	54	32.0	146	43.2
Pri-Occupation						
Farming own land/ sharecropper	61	36.8	40	24.0	101	30.3
Agriculture labourW	33	19.9	40	24.0	73	21.9
Non-agriculture labour	33	19.9	32	19.2	65	19.5
Fishing	3	1.8	15	9.0	18	5.4
Trade/Business	0	0.0	1	0.6	1	0.3
Self employed/petty business	1	0.6	2	1.2	3	0.9
House wife	11	6.6	15	9.0	26	7.8
Student	3	1.8	7	4.2	10	3.0
Unpaid family worker	2	1.2	4	2.4	6	1.8
White collar service	18	10.8	3	1.8	21	6.3
Not applicable/none	0	0.0	1	0.6	1	0.3
Others	1	0.6	7	4.2	8	2.4

More than 80 percent families in deltaic village and 66 percent families in non-deltaic village are nuclear families. And, more than 90 percent families in deltaic village and 88 percent families in non-deltaic village live in kutcha houses. On average, houses of more than 60 percent families live in one-room house in deltaic village and most of the families in non-deltaic village (51 percent) live in two-room house. Most of them either cook in the open terrace or outside the house under a roof made up of dry leaves and crop residue. Almost 100 percent families in both the villages use biomass fuel for cooking. Near about all of them use hand pump as water source, but 59 percent families in deltaic village and 69 percent families in non-deltaic village uses sanitary latrine for defecation. In deltaic village Krishnadaspur, 45 percent households have power where 68 percent families in non-deltaic village Rajrajeswarpur have it. Most of them in both the villages have solar power as a substitute of electricity. Most of the families in the study area do farming either in own land, do share cropping or work as agricultural labourer in others land. From qualitative study, it is evident that due to seasonal nature of agricultural work, they also engage themselves in works related to electrical wiring, construction work, fishing, and participate in Village Theater.

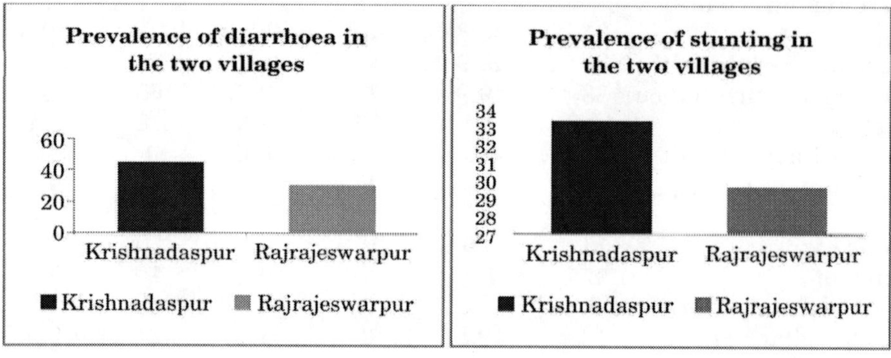

Figure 5.2: Prevalence of gastrointestinal problems and stunting in the study area

It is evident from the charts (Figure 5.2) that, prevalence of gastrointestinal problems and stunting is higher in deltaic village compared to non-deltaic village.

7

Impact of Climatic Shock

This chapter deals with impact of cyclones and floods on household assets, physical infrastructure of the villages and treatment seeking of children which the inhabitants are experiencing every year for a longer period of time. FGD with earning members in both the villages helped us to understand how they project the cyclones and become aware. Weather forecast in radio, frequent low pressure during rainy season, stormy wind from east – any of these make them aware about coming cyclones. With stormy wind from east, river water level increases and enters the village breaking the embankments and the village goes under water within an hour. Government and relief societies help during that period but still the initiatives are inadequate. During that time most of roads becomes inaccessible, no transport can move.

Child health deteriorates during the period of natural calamities. Since food becomes scarce adults can survive with only one meal a day with poor quality food but children cannot. Water becomes scarce and contaminated and they told about one event on drinking water supply during climatic shock.

Inhabitants of Krishnadaspur undergo sufferings due to climatic shock more compared to residents of Rajrajeswarpur village. Ninety six percent land and houses in deltaic village were completely devastated compared to non-deltaic village where the impact is visible on 83 percent households.

Table# 17 depicts the impact of climatic shock on household assets. We asked the households to rate the degree of impact on a four/five point scale – not at all, does not matter, very little, fairly/ more often, to a great extent. Ninety seven percent of deltaic village households and 83 percent of non-deltaic village households experienced great damage of housing, 84 percent of deltaic villagers lost their livestock to a great extent whereas 25 percent of non-deltaic villagers only suffer from such a deep impact. Land and/or crops of 58 percent deltaic villagers and 53 percent of non-deltaic villagers were damaged to a great extent. Drinking water source of 56.6 percent households in Krishnadaspur and 46.8 percent in Rajrajeswarpur was highly contaminated while lower degree of contamination is experienced by non-deltaic villagers (53.3 percent of non-deltaic villagers experienced very little or moderate degree of contamination whereas such degree of impact is visible among 43.4 percent households of deltaic village). When we asked about their perceptions about water contamination, household members said that after climatic shock drinking water coming from tube well become salty and muddy.

Table# 17: Impact of climatic shock on assets in last five years in the two GPs of the Patharpratima block

	G - Plot		***Ramganga***		***Total***	
	Krishnadaspur		***Rajrajeswarpur***			
	N	***%***	***N***	***%***	***N***	***%***
Whether land, house destroyed						
Devastated	157	95.7	140	82.8	297	89.2
No impact	0	0.0	1	0.6	1	0.3
Partially destroyed	7	4.3	28	16.6	35	10.5
Degree of impact on assets						
Housing						
Not at all	0	0.0	1	0.6	1	0.3
Very little	0	0.0	2	1.2	2	0.6
Fairly	5	3.0	26	15.4	31	9.3
To a great extent	161	97.0	140	82.8	301	89.9

Table# 17: (*Contd...*)

Table# 17: (*Contd...*)

	G - Plot		***Ramganga***		***Total***	
	Krishnadaspur		***Rajrajeswarpur***			
	N	*%*	***N***	*%*	***N***	*%*
Livestock						
Not at all	14	9.0	31	19.8	45	14.4
Very little	8	5.1	52	33.1	60	19.2
Fairly	50	32.1	35	22.3	85	27.2
To a great extent	84	53.9	39	24.8	123.0	39.3
Land/Crop						
Not at all	22	14.6	29	19.6	51	17.1
Very little	13	8.6	15	10.1	28	9.4
Fairly	28	18.5	25	16.9	53	17.7
To a great extent	88	58.3	79	53.4	167	55.9
Drinking water						
Not at all	9	5.4	5	3.0	14	4.2
Very little	20	12.1	28	16.6	48	14.3
Fairly	43	25.9	57	33.7	100	29.9
To a great extent	94	56.6	79	46.8	173	51.6
Impact on pri-occupation						
Land productive capacity is reducing						
Not at all	15	9.2	12	7.4	27	8.3
Does not matter	3	1.8	7	4.3	10	3.1
Very little	3	1.8	9	5.5	12	3.7
Fairly	62	38.0	71	43.6	133	40.8
To a great extent	80	49.1	64	39.3	144	44.2
Fishing become difficult						
Not at all	69	45.1	63	41.2	132	43.1
Does not matter	37	24.2	39	25.5	76	24.8
Very little	31	20.3	28	18.3	59	19.3
Fairly	14	9.2	15	9.8	29	9.5
To a great extent	2	1.3	8	5.2	10	3.3
Livestock rearing/honey collection/wood cutting becomes difficult						
Not at all	59	37.1	76	50.0	135	43.4
Does not matter	40	25.2	33	21.7	73	23.5
Very little	16	10.1	20	13.2	36	11.6
Fairly	25	15.7	18	11.8	43	13.8
To a great extent	19	12.0	5	3.3	24	7.7

Almost 50 percent of households in Krishnadaspur experienced decreasing land productivity to a greater degree, where more than 50 percent households earn their living by farming in own land, sharecropping or as agricultural labourers. In this manner, their livelihood becomes insecure with increase in salinity in agricultural land due to flood, and increase in barrenness due to draught. Such degree of impact is experienced by 39.3 percent households in Rajrajeswarpur. Mostly fishing was not or little affected as households argue that except during cyclone or flood fishing remains unaffected. Forty to fifty percent households informed that livestock rearing, honey collection not at all becomes difficult after climatic shock with the sense that though the roads approaching towards forest damage after climatic shock, they have no other option except honey collection or wood cutting. So 21.7 percent in non-deltaic village and 25.2 percent in deltaic village seems to be risk neutral. However, combating with chronic poverty with insecure livelihood to sustain their life trajectory they become resilient to the context and environment. Such insecure work opportunities and aggravated uncertainties due to climatic shock do not permit savings or asset accumulation (Begum and Sen, 2004). Therefore with limited agricultural produce and insecure livelihood, inhabitants fail to purchase required food for their family and such situation makes their children undernourished.

FGD with caregivers revealed that during flood, water comes inside their houses and destroys food storage so they remain without food for 2-3 days on average including children. Drinking water becomes scarce and water logging in the area pollutes the sources of drinking water supply. They told us that during "Aila" their houses and locality was under the water for 7-10 days. When the water drained out mud, decomposed fish and weeds inside the house polluted the environment a lot. Such environment makes children ill as during Aila[1] number of children under the age of five suffered from diarrhea and some of them died. Morbidity with

[1] The most remarkable thunder storm followed by devastating flood in 2009 among cumulative experiences for a long period of time.

water contamination and poor hygiene practice which gets aggravated after climatic events and such context increases the probability of under-nutrition severity (Mukherjee *et al.,* 2012).

Impact of Climatic Shock on Physical Accessibility in Krishnadaspur and Rajrajeswarpur

Table# 18 shows the impact of climatic shock on physical accessibility. In deltaic village, 52 percent households reported that village roads were damaged to a great extent while 51 percent households in non-deltaic village reported their village roads were damaged to some extent. Similarly, the impact on transport facility in deltaic village is higher compared to non-deltaic village as 45.8 percent households reported immense barrier in Krishnadaspur and 35.7 percent in Rajrajeswarpur. Service delivery in Government facility hampered to some extent in Krishnadaspur as reported by 44 percent of households. But in Rajrajeswarpur, most of them reported that impact on service delivery was very little. Most of the households in both the villages reported that climatic shock influenced physical access to schools very little. Regarding impact on telecommunication, most of the households in deltaic village reported that there was no impact. In relation to impact on service delivery of Government facility, access to school and telecommunication – a moderate percentage of households told that limited or no access to these public services does not matter. Qualitative survey reveals that, limited or no access to Government health facility leads to treatment seeking from rural healthcare provider, homeopath or traditional healer. With respect to physical access to schools, households were talking about Anganwadi centres since children under the age of five visit AWCs to receive elementary education as they are also supposed to get quality food every day. Those households reported that they have very poor experience regarding service delivery of AWCs – discrimination, supply of poor quality supplementary food, rough and aggressive behaviour of few anganwadi workers (AWW) – demotivate them to send their children to AWCs. Therefore it does

Table# 18: Impact of climatic shock on physical accessibility in the two GPs of the Patharpratima block

	G - Plot		*Ramganga*		*Total*	
	Krishnadaspur		*Rajrajeswarpur*			
	N	*%*	*N*	*%*	*N*	*%*
Degree of impact						
Village road						
Very little	0	0	16	9.5	16	4.8
Fairly	80	48.2	86	51.2	166	49.7
To a great extent	86	51.8	66	39.3	152	45.5
Condition of Transport						
Does not matter	4	2.4	1	0.6	5	1.5
Very little	24	14.5	39	23.2	63	18.9
Fairly	62	37.4	68	40.5	130	38.9
To a great extent	76	45.8	60	35.7	136	40.7
Service from Government health facility						
Not at all	6	3.6	11	6.6	17	5.1
Does not matter	29	17.5	30	18.0	59	17.7
Very little	35	21.1	52	31.1	87	26.1
Fairly	73	44.0	45	27.0	118	35.4
To a great extent	23	13.9	29	17.4	52	15.6
School						
Not at all	32	19.3	38	22.6	70	21.0
Does not matter	46	27.7	34	20.2	80	24.0
Very little	54	32.5	41	24.4	95	28.4
Fairly	31	18.7	30	17.9	61	18.3
To a great extent	3	1.8	25	14.9	28	8.4
Tele-communication						
Not at all	59	35.8	49	29.3	108	32.5
Does not matter	47	28.5	49	29.3	96	28.9
Very little	29	17.6	13	7.8	42	12.7
Fairly	27	16.4	21	12.6	48	14.5
To a great extent	3	1.8	35	21.0	38	11.5

not matter whether AWCs remain accessible during rainy season or during and after climatic shocks. Regarding telecommunication, the deltaic village does not have telecommunication network during even normal time. So it does not matter whether extreme climatic events took place or not. But in non-deltaic village, it does not matter because even if telecommunication was damaged, facility and centres are accessible with better roads and transports compared to deltaic village.

Impact of Climatic Shock on Child's Treatment Seeking in the Study Area

Table# 19 shows the impact of climatic shock on child's treatment seeking. Regarding impact of climatic shock on child's treatment seeking, we have asked whether Government facilities do not have or have limited human resource, transportation towards facility gets hampered, roads were damage or broken, shortage of medicines and equipments and increase in patient loads were experienced during shocks. In Krishnadaspur, reaction of 52

Table# 19: Impact of climatic shock on child treatment seeking in the two GPs of the Patharpratima block

	G - Plot		*Ramganga*		*Total*	
	Krishnadaspur		*Rajrajeswarpur*			
	N	*%*	*N*	*%*	*N*	*%*
Degree of impact						
No human resource at Govt. facility						
Not at all	21	13.6	40	26.3	61	19.9
Does not matter	18	11.7	25	16.5	43	14.1
Very little	5	3.3	17	11.2	22	7.2
Fairly	30	19.5	29	19.1	59	19.3
To a great extent	80	52.0	41	27.0	121	39.5
No transport facility						
Not at all	31	21.5	48	33.1	79	27.3
Does not matter	7	4.9	11	7.6	18	6.2
Very little	12	8.3	23	15.9	35	12.1
Fairly	35	24.3	29	20.0	64	22.2
To a great extent	59	41.0	34	23.5	93	32.2
Broken and damaged road						
Not at all	31	19.6	53	32.9	84	26.3
Does not matter	6	3.8	11	6.8	17	5.3
Very little	17	10.8	11	6.8	28	8.8
Fairly	46	29.1	40	24.8	86	27.0
To a great extent	58	36.7	46	28.6	104	32.6

Table# 19: (*Contd...*)

Table# 19: (*Contd...*)

	G - Plot		*Ramganga*		*Total*	
	Krishnadaspur		*Rajrajeswarpur*			
	N	*%*	*N*	*%*	*N*	*%*
Non-availability of medicine and equipments in hospitals						
Not at all	67	49.3	62	42.5	129	45.7
Does not matter	25	18.4	23	15.8	48	17.0
Very little	30	22.1	21	14.4	51	18.1
Fairly	13	9.6	22	15.1	35	12.4
To a great extent	1	0.7	18	12.3	19	6.7
Patient load in hospitals						
Not at all	71	52.6	70	49.0	141	50.7
Does not matter	27	20.0	30	21.0	57	20.5
Very little	29	21.5	16	11.2	45	16.2
Fairly	8	5.9	14	9.8	22	7.9
To a great extent	0	0.0	13	9.1	13	4.7

percent households was that they do not get any service delivery personnel in Government facility during climatic shock. Almost half of the interviewed households experienced the same degree of impact in Rajrajeswarpur. Problem of no or little transport facility is felt to a great extent during climatic shock is the experience of more than 40 percent households in deltaic village but such percentage is 23.5 in non-deltaic village. Damage of roads due to climatic events hindered child's health seeking to a great extent for 36.7 percent households in deltaic village while it is true for only 28.6 percent in non-deltaic village. Forty to fifty percent did not face shortage of medicines and equipments during climatic shock. Regarding patient load, 52.6 percent households in deltaic village and 49 percent households in non-deltaic village reported that patient load in Government facility does not increase during climatic shock as most of them visit rural unqualified providers in need of emergency or any care seeking. Though villages under study are selected on the basis of some prior information that differentiate them with respect to characteristics; detailed impact of climatic shock as above was never captured before which reflects how contextual uncertainty have differentiated impact on different geographic communities.

8

Under-Nutrition and Morbidity Among Children in the Study Area

In this chapter, I represent the prevalence of under-nutrition and morbidity by background characteristics of children. Background characteristics include household, mother and child level characteristics, and source of vulnerability. Along with these, other factors include five dimensions of access - *Acceptability, physical accessibility, affordability, accommodation and availability* (Balarajan *et al.*, 2011; IIHMR, 2010).

Influence of household, mother and child level characteristics: Table# 20 represents the influence of child's background characteristics on morbidity and nutritional status.

INFLUENCE ON PREVALENCE OF GASTROINTESTINAL PROBLEMS

Household Characteristics: Incidence of gastrointestinal problems in last fifteen days preceding the survey in deltaic village is higher in lower expenditure tercile, joint families, crowded houses, where source of cooking fuel is biomass fuel (mostly crop residues), families who do not have sanitary latrine, do not possess electricity, main source of income is in kind instead of cash, families of agricultural labourers, fishermen, and women headed families who perform only household works.

Table# 20: Influence of different household, mother and child level factors on child's ailments and nutritional status

Krishnadaspur			*Rajrajeswarpur*		
	Gastro enteric troubles	***Height for age compared to WHO growth standard***		***Gastro-enteric troubles***	***Height for age compared to WHO growth standard***
Household Characteristics	–	33.5	***Household Characteristics***	–	29.7
Monthly consumption expenditure	–		***Monthly consumption expenditure***	–	–
500-2000	57.9	31.6	500-2000	61.5	25.0
2001-3000	48.5	33.0	2001-3000	30.9	31.2
3000 & above	31.8	33.3	3000 & above	17.5	29.1
Family type			***Family type***		
Nuclear	43.8	31.3	Nuclear	38.9	27.9
Joint	50.0	43.3	Joint	14.3	33.3
House type			***House type***		
Kutcha	44.8	32.9	Kutcha	32.4	32.4
Semi-Pucca	42.9	42.9	Semi-Pucca	6.7	0.0
Pucca	50.0	37.5	Pucca	40.0	40.0
Number of rooms			***Number of rooms***		
1	45.1	34.0	1	33.9	26.4
2	45.9	32.2	2	33.7	31.7
More than 2	33.3	40.0	More than 2	12.5	30.4
Type of cooking fuel			***Type of cooking fuel***		
Wood	33.3	33.3	Wood	33.3	0.0
Crop residues	45.3	34.6	Crop residues	33.1	30.2
Cow dung cakes	25.0	0.0	Cow dung cakes	13.6	31.8
Liquid petroleum gas			Liquid petroleum gas	0.0	0.0
Drinking water source			***Drinking water source***		
Open well	0.0	0.0	Open well	0.0	0.0
Type of latrine			***Type of latrine***		
Sanitary latrine - Yes	42.0	35.4	Sanitary latrine - Yes	34.2	27.3
No	49.3	30.8	No	23.1	35.4

Table# 20: (*Contd...*)

Table# 20: (*Contd...*)

Krishnadaspur			***Rajrajeswarpur***		
	Gastro enteric troubles	***Height for age compared to WHO growth standard***		***Gastro-enteric troubles***	***Height for age compared to WHO growth standard***
Electricity			***Electricity***		
Yes	35.1	38.4	Yes	31.3	26.8
No	53.3	29.5	No	29.6	36.0
Pri-Occupation			***Pri-Occupation***		
Farming own land/sharecropper	42.6	30.0	Farming own land/ sharecropper	40.0	18.0
Agriculture labour	45.5	43.3	Agriculture labour	45.2	23.8
Non-agriculture labour	28.6	55.9	Non-agriculture labour	12.5	44.4
Fishing	66.7	0.0	Fishing	26.7	16.7
Self employed/ petty	100.0	0.0	Trade/Business	0.0	0.0
Home-based worker	36.4	0.0	Self employed/petty	50.0	50.0
Unemployed	33.3	33.3	Home-based worker	26.7	42.9
House wife	50.0	0.0	Unemployed	14.3	50.0
Unpaid family worker	83.3	18.8	House wife	0.0	50.0
Others	100.0	0.0	Unpaid family worker	33.3	33.3
			Not applicable/none	0.0	0.0
			Others	28.6	42.9
Mother's age			***Mother's age***		
13-19	44.4	50.0	13-19	28.6	53.8
20-25	47.6	33.0	20-25	27.4	34.6
26-30	40.4	34.8	26-30	44.2	18.0
31 & above	44.4	22.2	31 & above	10.5	23.5
Mother's education			***Mother's education***		
Illiterate	18.2	27.3	Illiterate	44.4	33.3
Literate	57.7	36.0	Literate	36.4	22.0
Up to Primary	50.7	34.4	Up to Primary	37.5	28.9
Higher	35.7	30.2	Higher	19.2	37.5

Table# 20: (*Contd...*)

Table# 20: (*Contd...*)

Krishnadaspur			*Rajrajeswarpur*		
	Gastro en-teric troubles	***Height for age compared to WHO growth standard***		***Gast-ro-en-teric troubles***	***Height for age compared to WHO growth standard***
Mother's nutritional status			***Mother's nutritional status***		
Underweight	51.3	26.3	Underweight	29.8	37.0
Normal	43.9	38.0	Normal	33.0	25.0
Overweight	42.9	28.6	Overweight	23.8	35.0
Mother's connection to health facility			***Mother's connection to health facility***		
Limited connection	56.7	29.6	Limited connection	42.4	23.7
Moderate connection	28.6	33.3	Moderate connection	24.4	30.2
Good connection	31.4	46.9	Good connection	20.0	36.7
Child delivered			***Child delivered***		
Before 6th month of pregnancy	41.2	33.3	Before 6th month of pregnancy	17.2	27.6
Before 7th month of pregnancy	46.0	34.3	Before 7th month of pregnancy	38.0	30.9
At 7th month	50.0	16.7	At 7th month	18.5	25.9
At 8th month	50.0	50.0	At 8th month	20.0	40.0
Child's age			***Child's age***		
0-5 months	33.3	50.0	0-5 months	20.0	50.0
6-11 months	23.1	46.1	6-11 months	21.7	40.9
12-23 months	48.7	32.4	12-23 months	28.1	38.7
24-35 months	53.9	50.0	24-35 months	33.3	33.3
36-59 months	44.7	26.5	36-59 months	36.2	19.1
Size of the child at birth			***Size of the child at birth***		
Small	48.3	37.0	Small	31.4	41.2
Medium	46.3	31.9	Medium	33.3	25.5

Table# 20: (*Contd...*)

Table# 20: *(Contd...)*

Krishnadaspur			*Rajrajeswarpur*		
	Gastro enteric troubles	***Height for age compared to WHO growth standard***		***Gastro-enteric troubles***	***Height for age compared to WHO growth standard***
Large	27.3	40.0	Large	23.1	33.3
Sex of the child			***Sex of the child***		
Girl	48.7	33.3	Girl	30.1	27.5
Boy	41.5	33.8	Boy	31.2	32.8
Place of delivery			***Place of delivery***		
Home	56.4	28.3	Home	42.7	22.9
Institution	30.7	40.6	Institution	22.8	34.0
Treatment seeking of child			***Treatment seeking of child***		
Government health facility	0.0	0.0	Government health facility	3.8	18.7
Private qualified provider	1.3	100.0	Private provider qualified	3.8	75.0
Quack/RMP	98.7	0.0	Quack/RMP	92.3	6.2

In non-deltaic village also households' monthly expenditure is negatively associated with gastrointestinal problems. Children living in nuclear families are more sufferers. This is mainly because, improper care of children as mothers are also involved in agriculture, knotting baskets, brooms etc for alternative employment as depicted from Focused Group Discussion of young mothers and caregivers. Surprisingly, children living in pucca houses are suffering more as evident in deltaic village. Similarly, here also children living in crowded families are suffering more. Households using unprocessed biomass fuels *e.g.,* wood, crop residue for cooking, earn through petty business, work as agricultural labourer, have sanitary latrine but do not follow proper hygiene practice show higher incidence of gastrointestinal problems during last fifteen days preceding the survey.

Mother's Characteristics: In delta region, incidence of gastrointestinal problems marginally varies by mother's age. But in non-delta region, children of middle aged (26-30 years) are suffering more. In delta region, children of literate or educated (up to primary level) mothers are suffering more compared to children of illiterate mothers. One reason is that sample contains higher percentage of mothers having children under the age of five within the age group of 26-30 years. But in non-deltaic village, children of illiterate mothers are suffering more. Not only questionable quality of primary education, but other contextual factors increase the vulnerability to be morbid in deltaic village. According to in depth interview of the key informant in deltaic village, physical inaccessibility due to geographical adversity is one main cause that retards the treatment seeking of children. Even they belong to educated family and understand the need of health seeking, they are unable to seek. In deltaic village children of undernourished mothers are suffering more. It proves that intergenerational transfer of under-nutrition is visible in inaccessible village Krishnadaspur implying existence of under-nutrition-morbidity vicious circle instead of the presence of ICDS centres and Sub Health Centres but nearby Primary Health Centre is in Indrapur which is 12-14 km far from Krishnadaspur takes minimum 1hour to reach there. As reported by mothers and caregivers, AWCs are ineffective with respect to service delivery though SHCs work properly especially in relation to ANC checkups of mothers and immunization of children. In non-deltaic village, prevalence of gastrointestinal problems varies marginally by mother's nutritional status. In both the villages if mother has limited connection with health provider her child suffers more. Quantitative study reveals that most of the children are delivered before expected delivery date. According to the view of one ICDS worker, it is because pregnant women do not eat properly and so the under-nutrition of the children starts from the womb. "*poatira khayna to bachhata peter bhitore barbe kikore*". Above 40 percent of children whether delivered at or before 6th month, 7th month or 8th month were suffering more from gastrointestinal problems. In non-deltaic village suffering is less than 20 percent among them.

Child Level Characteristics

In both deltaic and non-deltaic village, older children between the age group of 12-35 months are suffering most as they come to the contact of outside more compared to younger children. In the villages, children aged 36-59 months are suffering more. Though we cannot reach any conclusion about suffering distribution with respect to age since it is a cross-sectional study, to unveil the true picture, we need to conduct cohort or longitudinal study. Suffering is higher among children of small and medium size (at birth) in both the villages. Girl children are suffering more in deltaic village whereas in non-deltaic village there is marginal difference in suffering between them. In both the villages, children who are delivered at home and who generally seek treatment from unqualified provider, reporting of gastrointestinal problems is higher with respect to them and it is higher in deltaic village.

PREVALENCE OF STUNTING BASED ON WHO GROWTH STANDARD

Household Level Characteristics

In deltaic village, stunting is higher among children belonging to joint families, living in semi-pucca or pucca houses, houses with more than two rooms, families which use crop residue as cooking fuel, has sanitary latrine, have electricity, where earning members remain seasonally employed in agriculture or non-agricultural activities and unemployed in rest of the periods.

In non-deltaic village, stunting is higher among children of moderate poor families, joint families, living in pucca houses, houses with more than one room, families which use crop residue or cow dung as cooking fuel, do not have sanitary latrine, do not have electricity, where earning members works as casual labour in non-agricultural field or self–employed, home based workers or unemployed.

Mother Level Characteristics

In deltaic village, stunting is higher among children of teenage mothers, mothers who are not formally educated, who are normally nourished, and have good contact with health facility.

In non-deltaic village, stunting is higher among children of teenage mothers, educated mothers, underweight mothers, and have good contact with health service delivery.

Child Level Characteristics

In deltaic village, children who are delivered premature, aged under five months or 24-35 months, larger children, who are delivered at home, and seek treatment from private qualified providers are more stunted.

In non-deltaic village, children who are delivered premature, aged under the five months of age, smaller children, boys, delivered at institution and seek treatment from private qualified providers are more stunted.

Intergenerational transfer of under-nutrition is more in non-deltaic village. Along with this inaccessibility with respect to treatment seeking and child delivery is higher in deltaic village.

PHYSICAL ACCESSIBILITY, AFFORDABILITY, AVAILABILITY, ACCEPTABILITY AND ACCOMMODATION

Accessibility dimension from demand side perspective – 5 as – Acceptability, physical accessibility, affordability, accommodation and availability.

Table# 21: Perception about Accessibility from demand side in two villages of two GPs

	Krishnadaspur		***Rajrajeswarpur***	
	Prevalence of gastro-enteric troubles	***Height for age compared to WHO growth standard***	***Prevalence of gastro-enteric troubles***	***Height for age compared to WHO growth standard***
Social acceptability				
Delivery in the institution				
Not necessary	17.3	12.0	57.7	80.0
Family/husband did not allow	13.5	4.0	38.5	40.0
Better care at home	3.8	4.0	0.0	
No female doctor at hospital	0.0		0.0	
Nobody suggested	1.9		11.5	
Not customary	3.8	0.0	0.0	10.0
Not customary because angry ancestors will curse	0.0	0.0	0.0	0.0
Witchcraft from envious neighbours	0.0	0.0	0.0	0.0
Contaminate food with poison or other items to harm the baby	0.0	0.0	1.9	0.0
Treatment seeking				
RMP belongs to same religion and caste	–	–	–	–
Better than qualified doctor	4.0	2.0	14.3	7.5
Trust RMP	8.0	10.0	10.2	15.0
Visited in the past	20.0	28.0	16.3	27.5
Neighbours visited in the past	8.0	2.0	8.2	2.5
Accommodation				
Treatment seeking				
Always available	24.0	34.0	20.4	27.5
Provide treatment and medicine	2.7	6.0	2.0	5.0
Provide treatment and medicine on credit	22.7	34.0	12.2	25.0
Physical accessibility				

Table# 21: (*Contd...*)

Table# 21: *(Contd...)*

	Krishnadaspur		*Rajrajeswarpur*	
	Prevalence of gastro-enteric troubles	***Height for age compared to WHO growth standard***	***Prevalence of gastro-enteric troubles***	***Height for age compared to WHO growth standard***
Delivery in the institution				
No transport facility	63.5	84.0	7.7	30.0
Treatment seeking				
RMP clinic is nearby	84.0	70.0	77.5	57.5
No public facility nearby	0.0	0.0	2.0	2.5
Availability				
Delivery in the institution				
Health facility is too far	26.9	32.0	15.4	10.0
Treatment seeking				
Absence of doctor at public facility	4.0	6.0	6.1	0.0
No trained doctor nearby	28.0	24.0	14.3	17.5
Affordability				
Delivery in the institution				
Cost too high	57.7	24.0	84.6	60.0
Treatment seeking				
RMP services are less costly	22.7	10.0	38.8	27.5

Table# 21 represents the morbidity and under-nutrition of children in the study area by five dimensions of access.

Social Acceptability

Deltaic: Seventeen percent households with children suffering from gastrointestinal problems thinks institutional delivery is not necessary, 13.5 percent reported husband or family did not allow, 3.8 percent thinks family members attain better, and 4 percent said that it is not customary. With respect to treatment seeking of ailing children, 8 percent reported that they trust RMPs and 28 percent based on previous experience. Non-deltaic – Among households of under five children whose children were suffering from gastrointestinal problems fifteen days preceding the survey about 58 percent of them thinks institutional delivery is not necessary, 38.5 percent reported family or husband did not allow, regarding treatment seeking of children, 14.3 percent reported that RMPs are better than qualified providers, 10 percent of them visit due to their trust and 24.5 percent relies based on their own as well as neighbour's experience.

***Deltaic*:** In deltaic village, stunting is evident among families who think institutional delivery is not necessary (12 percent), where family or husband did not allow the respondent for institutional delivery (4 percent) and who thinks that mother and child get better care at home (4 percent). Prevalence is higher among children where respondents reported that they prefer RMPs for treatment seeking because of their good experience in the past (28 percent), trust RMP more than any other qualified provider (10 percent), and they perceives that RMPs are better than qualified providers (2 percent) with respect to behaviour and promptness.

***Non-Deltaic*:** Here stunting is evident among 80 percent families who believe that institutional delivery is not necessary. Forty percent respondents who reported that family or husband did not allow, have stunted children. Ten percent of respondents have stunted children who said that home delivery is customary. Here also respondents prefer RMPs for similar reasons – 27.5 percent reported they have better experience in the past, 15 percent prefers due to trust, 7.5 percent prefers due to perception in favour of them.

Accommodation

***Deltaic*:** In relation to treatment seeking of children who suffered from gastrointestinal problems fifteen days preceding the survey, 2.7 percent visit RMPs as they provide medicine along with treatment, and 22.7 percent said that they prefer because RMPs provide treatment and medicine on credit.

In non-deltaic village, 2 percent prefer them due to providing treatment and medicine and 12 percent prefer them due to provision of treatment and medicine on credit.

Stunting is higher among families who visit RMPs due to provision of service package (treatment and medicine) on credit in both the villages (34 percent in Krishnadaspur and 25 percent in Rajrajeswarpur).

Physical Accessibility

***Deltaic*:** Among families having morbid children during last fifteen days preceding the survey, 63.5 percent reported that there is no transport available when she was in need of the delivery of the child. Eighty four percent visit RMPs due to proximity. Mothers of 84 percent stunted children argue that non-availability of transport is the main cause of preferring home delivery of their children. Seventy percent mothers of stunted children prefer to seek treatment of their children from RMP due to proximity.

***Non-deltaic*:** In Rajrajeswarpur, 7.7 percent mothers of morbid children faced the problem of transport at the time of delivery, and 77.5 percent prefer treatment of their children in RMP's clinic due to closeness of the clinic from their house. Thirty percent mothers of stunted children delivered at home due to non-availability of transport and 57.5 percent prefer RMPs for proximity.

Availability

Twenty seven percent mothers of the morbid children, 32 percent mothers of the stunted children in the deltaic village reported that they prefer home delivery as distance from health facility is too long in the sense that distance is not much but it takes time due to poor road condition. In non-deltaic village, only 15.4 percent mothers of morbid children revealed their preference of home delivery due to time and distance factor. Twenty eight percent mothers of morbid children in deltaic village and 14.3 percent in non-deltaic village reported absence of trained doctor in nearby health facility. Four percent mothers of morbid children in deltaic village and 6 percent in non-deltaic village experience absence of doctors in public facility when they went for seeking treatment in public facility. In Krishnadaspur, 24 percent mothers of morbid children and 34 percent mothers of stunted children reported that they visit RMPs because they are always available. In non-deltaic village, 20 percent mothers of morbid children and 27.5 percent mothers of stunted children visit due to their easy availability. Thirty two percent mothers of stunted children in deltaic village compared to 10 percent in non-deltaic village preferred home delivery due to distance and time taken to reach health facility. Twenty four percent of the same reported that non-availability of trained doctor nearby in deltaic village compared to 17.5 percent in non-deltaic village.

Affordability

Among mothers of morbid children, 58 percent in deltaic village and 84.6 percent in non-deltaic village perceives institutional delivery is costly. Almost 23 percent of them in Krishnadaspur and 39 percent in Rajrajeswarpur reported RMP services are less costly. Twenty four percent mothers of stunted children in Krishnadaspur and 60 percent in Rajrajeswarpur perceives institutional delivery is costly. Ten percent mothers of stunted children in Krishnadaspur and 27.5 percent in Rajrajeswarpur reported that RMP services are less costly.

FGD with earning members in the villages revealed the people's perception which expressed that due to poor economic status, they are unable to take proper care of their children with respect to treatment seeking and other. Frequent climatic shock, geographical adversities induced physical inaccessibility, absence of qualified provider due to poor infrastructure, higher health expenditure on medicine due to lack of supply, and on transport due to unavailability of boat at night – all retards the care seeking even during emergency and so increases the likelihood of morbidity and further under-nutrition.

In summary, impact of social unacceptability is higher in non-deltaic village where availability of service package is more necessary in deltaic village. Impact of physical inaccessibility is higher in deltaic village where physical infrastructure gets destroyed more due to climatic shocks. Residents of remote areas in non-deltaic village prefer home delivery due to the same reason. Limited availability of service delivery affects mothers of stunted children more compared to those of morbid children to opt for home delivery and health seeking from unqualified provider. Affordability dimension is affecting the care giving of morbid children in non-deltaic village more compared to those in deltaic village or care giving of stunted children.

Effectiveness of Supply Side

In this chapter I analyzed how much the supply side environment is affecting the under-nutrition and morbidity of children in the study area.

Most of the households in both the villages seek treatment for their children from unqualified providers. The percentage sought treatment from unqualified providers is 80 percent in Krishnadaspur while 67 percent in Rajrajeswarpur. About treatment seeking of their children, approximately, 1 percent households went to PHC, 19.4 percent in Krishnadaspur and 27.9 percent in Rajrajeswarpur sought from SHC, 2.2 percent in Krishnadaspur and 11.4 percent in 2.2 percent in Rajrajeswarpur sought from homeopath, 2.2 percent in Krishnadaspur and 5 percent in Rajrajeswarpur went to BPHC and 0.7 percent in krishnadaspur went to DH.

Table# 22 shows the effectiveness of supply side environment during climatic shock. We asked the households whether cost of treatment increases during climatic shock in the clinic of unqualified provider. Thirty five percent of them in Krishnadaspur

Table# 22: Effectiveness of Supply side environment under climatic shock in two villages of two GPs

	G Plot		***Ramganga***		***Total***	
	Krishnadaspur		***Rajrajeswarpur***			
	N	***%***	***N***	***%***	***N***	***%***
Treatment seeking during emergency						
PHC	1	0.7	2	1.4	3	1.1
SHC	27	19.4	39	27.9	66	23.7
RMP	111	79.9	94	67.1	205	73.5
Alternative medicine	3	2.2	16	11.4	19	6.8
BPHC	3	2.2	7	5.0	10	3.6
DH	1	0.7	0	0.0	1	0.4
Other	3	2.2	3	2.1	6	2.2
Cost for treatment in RMP clinic during climatic shock increases						
Not at all	25	15.4	43	25.9	68	20.7
Sometimes	57	35.2	67	40.4	124	37.8
More often	51	31.5	45	27.1	96	29.3
To a great extent	29	17.9	11	6.6	40	12.2
Cost for treatment in any clinic due to						
Doctor	58	36.3	96	66.2	154	50.5
Medicine and test	88	55	71	49.0	159	52.1
Transport	13	8.1	13.0	9.0	26	8.5
Food, lodging	41	25.6	17	11.7	58	19.0

and 40.4 percent of them in Rajrajeswarpur reported that RMPs[1] sometimes charge more during extreme climatic events. In krishnadaspur, about 31.5 percent experienced cost increase frequently whereas in Rajrajeswarpur it is 27 percent. Experience of cost increase to a great extent due to seeking treatment of children from RMP's clinic is much higher in krishnadaspur (17.9 percent) compared to Rajrajeswarpur (6.6 percent). We also asked in what field households incurred expenditure due to treatment seeking of their children. *i.e.,* out of pocket expenditure for healthcare[2] Most of the households in Krishnadaspur (55 percent)

[1] RMP stands for rural medical practitioners who practice allopathic treatment without medical degree.

[2] It involves cost incurred during treatment seeking due to medicines, diagnostic test and transport.

incurred cost to purchase medicines and to do diagnostic tests and in Rajrajeswarpur, most of them incurred cost to pay doctor's visit (66.2 percent). The second most item in Krishnadaspur is doctor's fees and Rajrajeswarpur is purchase of medicines and tests.

Table# 23 shows the ICDS effectiveness. Exploring the impact of ICDS programme, it is evident that visit of AWW is lower in

Table# 23: ICDS effectiveness in the two villages in two GPs of the Patharpratima block

	G Plot		*Ramganga*		*Total*	
	Krishnadaspur		*Rajrajeswarpur*			
	N	*%*	*N*	*%*	*N*	*%*
Effectiveness of ICDS						
AWW visit						
Yes	120	75.9	113	68.5	239	72.2
No	40	24.1	52	31.5	92	27.8
Frequency of visit						
Weekly	0	0.0	2	1.7	2	0.8
Fortnightly	5	4.0	6	5.0	11	4.5
Monthly	73	58.4	65	54.2	138	56.3
Once in two months	47	37.6	47	39.2	94	38.4
Receive food from AWC						
Everyday	129	77.3	95	57.9	224	67.7
Weekly	15	9.0	26	15.9	41	12.4
Fortnightly	1	0.6	3	1.8	4	1.2
Monthly	0	0.0	1	0.6	1	0.3
Never give my child that food	5	3.0	15	9.2	20	6.0
Does not go to collect	10	6.0	16	9.8	26	7.9
Not given	7	4.2	8	4.9	15	4.5
Food sharing at home						
With none	7	4.9	9	7.7	16	6.2
With another one	81	57.0	53	45.3	134	51.7
With more than one	54	38.0	55	47.0	109	42.1
Food insecurity during climatic shock						
Not at all	32	19.5	45	28.0	77	23.7
Sometimes	53	32.3	63	39.1	116	35.7
More often	59	36.0	46	28.6	105	32.3
Toa great extent	20	12.2	7	4.4	27	8.3

Rajrajeswarpur (68.5 percent) compared to Krishnadaspur (75.9 percent). AWWs visit monthly or once in two months (58.4 percent in Krishnadaspur and 54.2 percent in Rajrajeswarpur). Receiving supplementary nutrition from AWC everyday is higher in Krishnadaspur (77.3 percent) than in Rajrajeswarpur (57.9 percent). Supplementary food sharing within more than three household members is higher in Rajrajeswarpur (47 percent against 38 percent) compared to Krishnadaspur where food sharing is higher between two members (57 percent against 45.3 percent). With regard to mother's perception regarding whether gathering of child's food becomes difficult during climatic shock, it is evident that in Rajrajeswarpur most of them perceives that they felt not at all (28 percent against 19.5 percent in Krishnadaspur) or sometimes (39.1 percent compared to 32.3 percent in Krishnadaspur). Forty eight percent of them in Krishnadaspur perceive the degree of impact is felt more often or to a great extent than 33 percent in Rajrajeswarpur.

Table# 24 represents morbidity and under-nutrition of children by ICDS effectiveness. In deltaic village, prevalence of gastro-enteric problems (42.9 percent) is higher among children where no visit by AWW takes place, frequency of AWW visit is once in two months (55.3 percent), and who receive food from AWC weekly (73.3 percent). But prevalence of stunting (37.8 percent) is higher among children where AWW visits once in a month (39.7 percent), and caregivers do not allow the baby to eat the food supplied from ICDS even if they collect (75 percent). We also asked whether the food collected from AWC is shared between others and we found that where the food is shared with more than one child or two, prevalence of gastro-enteric problems (61.1 percent) or stunting (41.6 percent) is higher among them. Higher percentage of gastrointestinal morbidity is visible among households who more often face food insecurity due to climatic shock compared to others (59.3 percent). Stunting is higher among them who not at all perceive any food insecurity due to climatic shock (51.7 percent).

Table# 24: Influence of ICDS ineffectiveness on childhood morbidity and undernutrition in the study area

Krishna-daspur	***Gast-ro en-teric trou-bles***	***Heig-ht for age comp-ared to WHO growth stan-dard***	***Rajrajesw-arpur***	***Gast-ro en-teric trou-bles***	***Height for age comp-ared to WHO growth stand-ard***
Effectiveness of ICDS			***Effectiveness of ICDS***		
AWW visit			***AWW visit***		
Yes	42.9	37.8	Yes	22.1	33.0
No	50.0	20.5	No	48.1	22.9
Frequency of visit			***Frequency of visit***		
Weekly	0.0	0.0	Weekly	0.0	0.0
Fortnightly	40.0	20.0	Fortnightly	0.0	0.0
Monthly	37.0	39.7	Monthly	20.0	36.5
Once in two months	55.3	34.8	Once in two months	31.9	30.9
Receive food from AWC			***Receive food from AWC***		
Everyday	44.2	31.7	Everyday	0.0	31.9
Weekly	73.3	40.0	Weekly	0.0	34.6
Fortnightly	0.0	100.0	Fortnightly	0.0	0.0
Monthly	0.0	0.0	Monthly	0.0	0.0
Never give my child that food	40.0	75.0	Never give my child that food	26.7	21.4
Does not go to collect	50.0	20.0	Does not go to collect	25.0	30.8
Not given	14.3	33.3	Not given	25.0	16.7
Food sharing at home			***Food sharing at home***		
With none	42.9	14.3	With none	22.2	28.6
With another one	35.8	41.6	With another one	18.9	46.0
With more than one	61.1	26.9	With more than one	49.1	24.1
Food insecurity during climatic shock			***Food insecurity during climatic shock***		
Not at all	40.6	51.7	Not at all	20.0	45.0
Sometimes	41.5	35.3	Sometimes	19.0	24.1
More often	59.3	17.5	More often	60.9	23.9
To a great extent	30.0	47.4	To a great extent	28.6	14.3

In non-deltaic village, gastrointestinal morbidity is higher among children where AWWs do not visit (48.1 percent), visit once in two months (31.9 percent), households never allow children to eat that food (26.7 percent), food is shared between more than two children/person (49.1 percent), and where mothers perceive that they more often face food insecurity due to climatic shock (60.9m percent). Stunting is higher among children where AWW visits (33 percent), visits monthly (36.5 percent), does not go to collect food from AWC (30.8 percent), food is shared with one child/person (46 percent), and where mothers perceive that they not at all face food insecurity during climatic shock (45 percent).

According to focused group discussion, provision of supplementary food is not provided in similar quality and frequency in all the centres. Caregivers said that one centre provides egg with khichdi three times a week whereas another provides less but the quality of khichdi is very poor.

The in depth-interview of anganwadi worker in Rajrajeswarpur village reveals the fact that though they are trying hard to generate awareness inside the community, responses are heterogeneous in nature. They teach about how to prepare the food, when to start complementary feeding, the frequency of feeding but mothers use very less quantity of ingredients to cook and so the food becomes nutrient deficient. Though mothers are educated to a certain level, they mostly go outside with other family members to reap or harvest paddy or knot baskets/brooms as alternate livelihoods which affect their childcare and feeding.

According to her, under-nutrition starts from the womb as intra-household food allocation disfavors the younger daughter-in-laws. Most of them suffer from reproductive morbidities and no treatment seeking hampers intrauterine growth of the children. Mothers are unable to produce breast milk enough as they drink very little quantity of milk and they hardly follow the norm of drinking water before or after breastfeeding. So even though they exclusively breastfed their children for first six months, the children are undernourished.

She said that view of beneficiaries of ICDS regarding its effectiveness is difficult to change. She argues that due to poor SES, people expect that ICDS support 24 × 7 is required but they do not understand that ICDS is designed to serve a part and rest of the care and feeding is to be done at home. Her suggestion to increase the effectiveness, she needs co-operation from NGOs and CBOs to increase the care during pregnancy and lactation period through proper intervention and monitoring otherwise child health and nutritional status cannot be improved.

Focused group discussion with caregivers revealed that in Krishnadaspur, children living in hard to reach parts are unable to go to AWCs to eat the supplementary food - khichdi. FGD with earning members in Rajrajeswarpur and caregivers in Krishnadaspur expressed high level of frustration about the questionable quality of supplementary food. They said that in khichdi, rice and pulse remains very little and not boiled properly, egg is provided once in a week ("*chal dal sidhho hoy na, ektufota thake, dim to sat dine ekdin dey*"). In Krishnadaspur, they are satisfied with the supplementary nutrition provided by SSDC. The caregivers in hard to reach areas raised the need for more AWW; all of them in both the villages want diligent workers to serve effectively so that every child can get service.

9

Community Perception and Involvement

This chapter explores how much community members feel for other members, their togetherness and interest to accomplish collective goals. These factors are important because community led interventions and solutions can better improve the scenario as solution from within the community level is always contextual compared to centrally driven strategies. Since, child health and nutrition problem related solution should count every child so individual level intervention will accelerate the reduction of inequity much faster compared to average based solutions.

As per key informant interview in the two villages – in Krishnadaspur, he strongly agrees with the view that if the community faces a collective problem, members can develop and carry out solutions to the problem when it arises. Because, this community has good mechanism to gather together and discuss problems the community is facing and most of the community members are trustworthy. He firmly agrees with the view that all the members are committed to same collective goals, people even women and the poor with differing views are able to equally contribute their views on community plans and activities. But as per Focused Group Discussions with mothers and earning members it is highlighted that young mothers are unable to take decisions about their children's health and nutrition due to disempowerment and hardly anybody or group listen to the poor as mentioned regarding the quality of supplementary food supplied by AWCs. The village leader also agrees to the view that the people in the community share similar ideas of what is best for the community members and community leaders represent the interest of the poor people and women. He disagrees with the view that the community frequently evaluates how well plans and projects have worked. He also disagrees with the view that people are self-centred, thinks only about their own interest or are not concerned with the larger community. In addition to this, he strongly disagrees that people in this community have poor skills and resources compared to other communities.

In Rajrajeswarpur, he strongly agrees that this community is committed to collective goals, community members develop and solve any problem the community faces, public institutions with participation of community frequently evaluates how well plans and projects have worked, community people are trustworthy. He also strongly argues that people in this community look out more for their own interest and less concerned about the interest of the poor people and women. He agrees with the view that when the community faces any problem, these community members gather together and discuss the solutions and poor people in this community are equally able to contribute their views and opinions on community plans and activities. But he disagrees with the view that women has equal voice on community matters and strongly disagrees with the view that community members share similar ideas regarding the best of the community.

To understand how much the community is responsive to child health seeking needs during climatic shock as well as normal time, it is evident from Figure 5.3 that families of morbid children who required treatment during gastrointestinal episodes, 39.5 percent of them in Krishnadaspur and 15.7 percent in Rajrajeswarpur reported that neighbours do not help regarding treatment seeking during climatic shock. Almost 40 percent households in Krishnadaspur and 20 percent in Rajrajeswarpur stated that they do not get any help during normal time also. Forty six percent in

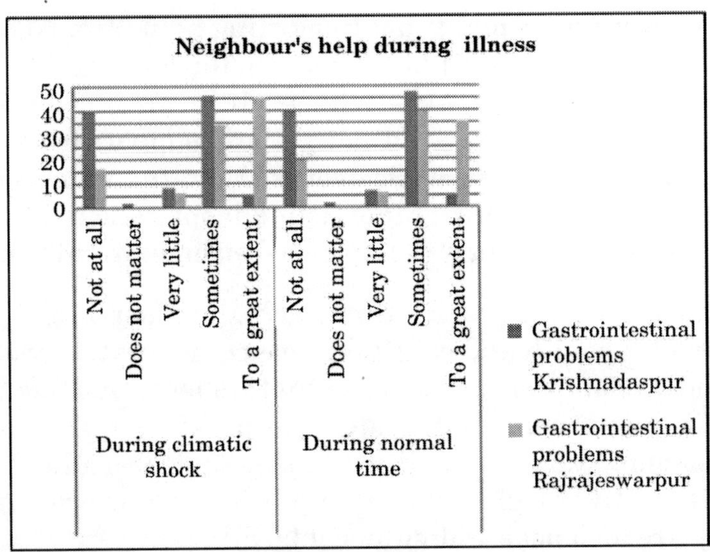

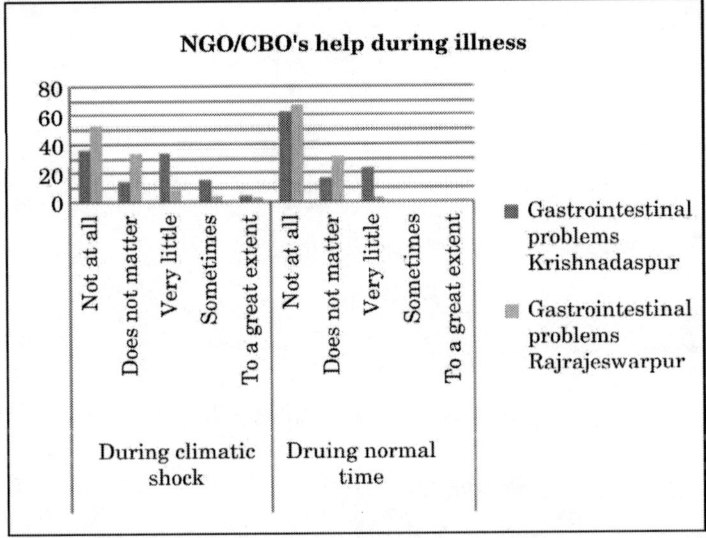

Figure 5.3: Community participation regarding treatment seeking of children during climatic shock as well as normal time in the study area

Krishnadaspur and 33.5 percent in Rajrajeswarpur sometimes get help from neighbours during climatic shock. Forty seven percent in Krishnadaspur and 39 percent in Rajrajeswarpur sometimes get support during normal time. Regarding help from NGOs and CBOs, more than 50 percent households in Rajrajeswarpur and 35 percent in Krishnadaspur – whose children suffered from gastrointestinal problems – did not get any support from NGOs/CBOs during periods of climatic events. More than 60 percent of such households (61.8 percent in Krishnadaspur and 66.7 percent in Rajrajeswarpur) do not get help even during normal time.

Qualitative study revealed that in Krishnadaspur one NGO – SSDC provides health and nutrition service, generates awareness about childcare and serves during climatic shock. But side by side it is difficult for them to provide care provider during all the episodes of emergency. In addition to this they also added that it is difficult for the neighbours to help in person or economically since they are also poor and vulnerable.

10

Poverty Dynamics, Under-Nutrition and Morbidity

This chapter explores the SES and morbidity linkage as well as SES – under-nutrition linkage. Not only SES, it also explores how vulnerability to future poverty, perception about vulnerability, perception about SES trend and actual deepening of poverty is linked to morbidity and under-nutrition.

Table# 25 represents impact of treatment seeking under climatic shock leading to poverty deepening. Ninety to ninety five percent respondents in both the villages experienced increase in healthcare expenditure during climatic shock at varying degrees. In deltaic village, 36.8 percent experienced more often increase and 33.7 percent reports increase to a great extent, 24.5 percent said they experienced but infrequently. In non-deltaic village, degree of impact differs from deltaic village. In Rajrajeswarpur, most of them (40 percent) experienced occasional increase, 32.3 percent reported more often increase, and at the same time, only 17.4 percent experienced increase to a great extent.

Ninety percent families in Krishnadaspur perceive economic status deterioration due to increase in healthcare expenditure during extreme climatic events for treatment seeking of their children. In Rajrajeswarpur, 82 percent such families perceive so but also in varying degrees. In deltaic village, 39 percent perceives that they experience more often and 32.3 percent perceives such

Table# 25: Impact of treatment seeking under climatic shock in two villages of two GPs leading to poverty deepening

	G Plot		*Ramganga*		*Total*	
	Krishnadaspur		*Rajrajeswarpur*			
	N	*%*	*N*	*%*	*N*	*%*
Expenditure on treatment seeking increases during climatic shock						
Not at all	8	4.9	16	10.3	24	7.6
Sometimes	40	24.5	62	40.0	102	32.1
More often	60	36.8	50	32.3	110	34.6
To a great extent	55	33.7	27	17.4	82	25.8
Perceived Economic status fall						
Not at all	14	8.7	28	18.2	42	13.3
Sometimes	32	19.9	64	41.6	96	30.5
More often	63	39.1	41	26.6	104	33.0
To a great extent	52	32.3	21	13.6	73	23.2
Consumption sacrifice						
Food	128	85.3	103	74.6	231	80.2
Treatment of other family member	42	28	32	23.2	74	25.7
School education	12	8	21	15.2	33	11.5
Social festivals	13	8.7	27	19.6	40	13.9
Purchase of durables	23	15.3	19	13.8	42	14.6
Repairing of assets, house	21	14	23	16.7	44	15.3
Actual Economic status fall						
Most poor with severe fall	34	23.0	33	23.6	67	23.3
Medium poor with moderate fall	81	54.7	69	49.3	150	52.1
Less poor with moderate fall	33	22.3	38	27.1	71	24.6

experience is congregated to a great extent. But only 13 percent of Rajrajeswarpur households experienced status fall to a great extent. Most of the households in non-deltaic village (40 percent) perceive occasional experience of status fall where such perception about the degree of impact is only among 19.9 percent households in deltaic village.

POVERTY→UNDER-NUTRITION AND MORBIDITY→ VULNERABILITY TO POVERTY

Table# 26 represents poverty dynamics, child's ailment and under-nutrition in the study area. Thirty eight percent children from most poor families in Krishnadaspur and 32 percent such children in Rajrajeswarpur suffered from gastrointestinal problems. It is higher among medium poor families, households who are experiencing poverty deepening through oscillated declining pattern of monthly expenditure away from the poverty line in the last five years, who do not perceive that their economic status deteriorates after treatment seeking during climatic shock in deltaic village. But if we study with respect to actual economic status fall, it is evident that moderate poor with moderate fall in economic status families reported higher prevalence of gastrointestinal problems in Krishnadaspur. In addition to this, 56.4 percent families among them experienced great extent of increase in expenditure on treatment seeking during climatic shock reported gastrointestinal problems among their children. On the contrary, 62.5 percent of families who experienced no increase in expenditure due to treatment seeking during climatic shock also reported children's gastrointestinal problems.

Stunting is higher among families who perceives healthcare expenditure increases during climatic shock sometimes (46.1 percent), who perceives that their economic status not at all deteriorates after healthcare spending (57.1 percent), where most poor families experienced severe economic status fall actually (36.4 percent), but among least poor families as per perception of economic status (39.6 percent) and families who are experiencing smooth or oscillated movement towards poverty line (50 percent)[1].

Focused Group Discussions with mothers and earning members reveal that during climatic shock their expenditure does not

[1]In this context, stunting is the dependent variable and economic status fall due to out of pocket spending is the independent variable and bivariate result is statistically significant.

Table# 26: Poverty dynamics and child's ailment, undernutrition in the two GPs

	Krishnadaspur		*Rajrajeswarpur*	
	Prevalence of Gastrointestinal problems	***Stunted compared to WHO reference population***	***Prevalence of Gastrointestinal problems***	***Stunted compared to WHO reference population***
Expenditure on treatment seeking increases during climatic shock				
Not at all	62.5	25.0	12.5	6.7
Sometimes	35.0	46.1	25.8	23.7
More often	40.0	33.9	38.0	27.7
To a great extent	56.4	24.5	37.0	60.0
Perceived Economic status fall				
Not at all	64.3	57.1	17.9	24.0
Sometimes	31.2	46.9	20.3	27.1
More often	39.7	30.5	48.8	31.7
To a great extent	57.7	20.4	42.9	40.0
Actual Economic status fall				
Most poor with severe fall	41.2	36.4	48.5	26.7
Medium poor with moderate fall	50.6	28.6	31.9	35.4
Less poor with moderate fall	33.3	29.0	21.0	21.0
Perceived Poverty				
Most Poor	38.2	29.6	32.1	35.2
Medium	53.6	34.6	38.6	30.2
Least Poor	39.6	39.1	16.7	23.3
Trajectory of Poverty perception				
Smooth pattern of chronic poverty	33.3	30.0	42.9	14.3
Smooth movement towards poverty line	57.1	50.0	14.3	50.0
Oscillated deepening of chronic poverty (declining saw-tooth)	58.0	20.8	39.1	27.7
Smooth abrupt deepening of chronic poverty	41.4	27.6	20.0	36.8
Gradual deepening of chronic poverty	40.4	48.8	25.0	39.1
Oscillated movement towards poverty line (improving saw-tooth)	27.3	50.0	13.6	21.1

increase – it never means that they are receiving effective service from existing Government facility or relief measures. But they argue that they first try with home remedies as access to facility becomes difficult. Then if situation worsens they take the help from local unqualified practitioners. However, when the area is blocked with water, it also becomes difficult for them to supply ORS and necessary medicines. So, sometimes morbid children do not get any medicine for cure even if they seek treatment. So not only availability and proximity of care provider is necessary, assurance of ORS and medicine supplies in those areas are important especially during or after climatic shock. Absence of which increases the vulnerability of children to be caught under under-nutrition-morbidity vicious circle and deepening of under-nutrition severity given the already proven example of intergenerational transfer of under-nutrition. Again where medicines and remedies are available, the cost of care increases. Such cost increase within family demotivates households to seek care further.

Non-deltaic- Reporting of gastrointestinal problems prevalence is higher among medium poor families, who perceives that they do not experience consumption volatility for last five years, higher among most poor with severe economic status fall, higher among families who experienced increase in healthcare expenditure more often or to a great extent during climatic shock and due to that who perceives economic status deterioration is moderate or high. Percentage of reporting of higher gastrointestinal problems prevalence is also higher among families who experience consumption decline with oscillated pattern of movement of economic status in last 5 years.

Stunting is higher among families who perceives healthcare expenditure increases during climatic shock to a great extent (60 percent), who perceives that their economic status deteriorates to a great extent after healthcare spending (40 percent), where medium poor families experienced moderate economic status fall actually (35.4 percent), but among most poor families as per perception of economic status (35.2 percent) and who are experiencing smooth movement of their economic status towards poverty line *i.e.*, lowering of poverty deepening.

IMPACT OF HEALTHCARE SPENDING LEADING TO POVERTY DEEPENING DURING CLIMATIC SHOCK

In order to meet healthcare expenditure during climatic shock, households of both the villages mostly sacrificed food consumption which is higher in deltaic village (85.3 percent in Krishnadaspur and 74.6 percent in Rajrajeswarpur). Sacrifice of treatment seeking of other family members and purchase of durable assets are also higher in Krishnadaspur (28 percent and 15.3 percents respectively sacrificed the said service and purchase). Other sacrifices like school education of children, repairing of houses or assets, social festivals are higher in non-deltaic village.

Percentage of households experiencing actual economic status fall due to healthcare expenditure in general, is also higher in deltaic village. Percentage of medium poor with moderate degree of economic status fall is higher in both areas with higher percentage in Krishnadaspur.

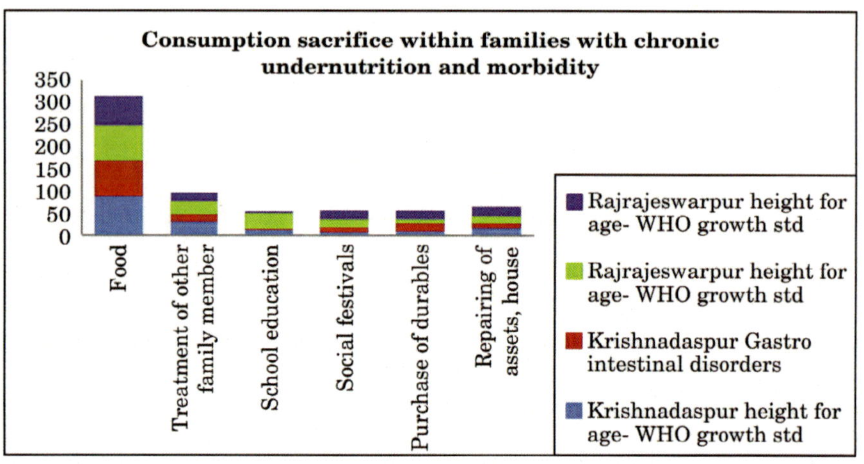

Figure 5.4: Consumption sacrifice after treatment seeking in the study area

Food consumption sacrifice (Figure 5.4) is higher among children with gastrointestinal problems in Krishnadaspur (86.6 percent). Next is the food sacrifice among families whose children are stunted in that village (81.8 percent). Percentage of households did food sacrifice whether having one stunted or morbid child is lower in Rajrajeswarpur. Among other sacrifices, treatment of others (30.4 percent) and school education of children (34.8 percent) are higher in Rajrajeswarpur families where children were suffering from gastrointestinal disorders.

In the FGD of caregivers and earning members, they all agree that their family generally run under deficit usually. Treatment seeking from qualified private provider in Rajrajeswarpur leads to food sacrifice more compared to villagers in Krishnadaspur as they generally seek treatment from RMPs. But who produce in their own land and store crops, they sacrifice less though they are very few in number.

11

Caregivers Perception, and Practice in the Study Area

This chapter analyses the perception of the mothers and grandmothers, practice about childcare and feeding in the two villages in the study area since these factors are important influencing factors determining childhood nutritional outcomes. Table# 27 shows the perception, and practice of child care in the study area. Most of the mothers in deltaic as well as non-deltaic village perceive their children are moderately healthy (55.4 percent in Krishnadaspur, 72.1 percent in Rajrajeswarpur). More than 80 percent of children were exclusively breastfed for first six months of life. Most children were started solid complementary feeding with stopping the breast milk (59.5 percent in Krishnadaspur and 57.5 percent in Rajrajeswarpur). Most of them are fed thrice daily (45.5 percent in Krishnadaspur and 48.3 percent in Rajrajeswarpur).

Table# 28 represents the morbidity and under-nutrition of children by mother's perception, and practice in the study area. Mothers who perceive their children are very healthy, 80 percent of them in deltaic village were suffering from gastrointestinal problems. Next are the children whose mothers perceive that their children are undernourished and suffer from ailments - 46 percent of them in deltaic village and 35.1 percent of them in non-deltaic village were suffering. They are the maximum sufferer in non-deltaic village. Suffering in deltaic village is higher among children

Table# 27: Mother's perception, practice in the study area

	G - Plot		***Ramganga***		***Total***	
	Krishnadaspur		***Rajrajeswarpur***			
	N	***%***	***N***	***%***	***N***	***%***
Perception about child's health and nutritional status						
Yes, very healthy	5	3.0	1	0.6	6	1.8
Moderate	93	55.4	119	72.1	212	63.7
Undernourished, suffer from ailments	63	37.5	37	22.4	100	30.0
Undernourished, but suffer less	7	4.2	8	4.9	15	4.5
Exclusive breastfeeding for first 6 months						
Yes	148	88.6	152	90	300	89.3
No	19	11.4	17	10.1	36	10.7
Nature of complementary feeding						
Semi-solid with breat milk	43	26.4	22	13.5	65	20.1
Semi-solid without breast milk	2	1.2	8	5	10	3.1
Solid with breast milk	15	9.2	12	7.5	27	8.4
Solid without breast milk	97	59.5	92	57.5	189	58.5
Not yet, only breast milk	6	3.7	22	13.7	28	8.7
Not yet, only other milk	0	0	4	2.5	4	1.2
Frequency of feeding						
Once	4	2.4	1	0.6	5	1.5
Twice	14	8.5	20	12.5	34	10.5
Thrice	75	45.5	82	51.3	157	48.3
Four times	61	37.0	44	27.5	105	32.3
More	11	6.7	13	8.1	24	7.4

who were not exclusively breastfed for first six months (52.6 percent), who were started semi-solid complementary food stopping the breast milk (100 percent), fed only once in a day (100 percent). In non-deltaic village evidence of higher suffering is prominent among children who were not exclusively breastfed for first six months (32.9 percent), were started semi-solid complementary food stopping the breast milk (37.5 percent), and

Table# 28: Influence of Mother's perception, practice on child's morbidity and undernutrition in the study area

Krishnadaspur	*Prevalence of gastroenteric troubles*	*Height for age as per WHO growth standard*	*Rajrajeswarpur*	*Prevalence of gastroenteric troubles*	*Height for age as per WHO growth standard*
Perception about child's health and nutriton status			***Perception about child's health and nutriton status***		
Yes, very healthy	80.0	40.0	Yes, very healthy	0.0	0.0
Moderate	42.0	45.0	Moderate	30.2	27.3
Undernourished, suffer from ailments	46.0	15.5	Undernourished, suffer from ailments	35.1	37.8
Undernouris hed, but suffer less	42.9	16.7	Undernourished, but suffer less	12.5	42.9
Exclusive breastfeeding for first 6 months			***Exclusive breastfeeding for first 6 months***		
Yes	44.6	34.7	Yes	32.9	28.9
No	52.6	27.8	No	11.8	37.5
Nature of complementary feeding			***Nature of complementary feeding***		
Semi-solid with breast milk	44.2	50.0	Semi-solid with breast milk	18.2	40.0
Semi-solid without breast milk	100.0	0.0	Semi-solid without breast milk	37.5	50.0
Solid with breast milk	40.0	15.4	Solid with breast milk	33.3	33.3
Solid without breast milk	45.4	30.5	Solid without breast milk	38.0	20.9
Not yet, only breast milk	33.3	33.3	Not yet, only breast milk	13.6	52.9
Not yet, only other milk	–	–	Not yet, only other milk	25.0	33.3
Frequency of feeding			***Frequency of feeding***		
Once	100.0	25.0	Once	0.0	0.0
Twice	28.6	53.9	Twice	10.0	57.9
Thrice	49.3	33.3	Thrice	32.9	30.4
Four times	41.0	30.0	Four times	36.4	16.3
More	45.4	33.3	More	38.5	27.3

surprisingly among children who were fed more than four times in a day (38.5 percent).

Stunting prevalence in deltaic village is higher among children, whose mothers perceive that their children are moderately healthy (45 percent), were exclusively breastfed for first six months (34.7 percent), were started semi-solid complementary food and are continuing breast milk (50 percent), and where frequency of feeding is twice in a day (53.9 percent). In non-deltaic village, stunting prevalence is higher among children whose mothers perceive that they are undernourished but suffer less (42.9 percent), were not exclusively breastfed for first six months (37.5 percent), were not started complementary food and are only breast fed (50 percent), or eating more than four times a day (52.9 percent).

The stunting prevalence is influenced also by early child bearing, caregiver's perception about child's health and nutritional status and the feeding practice.

Qualitative study reflects the care giving practice of the study area. In Krishnadaspur and Rajrajeswarpur village, the FGD with caregivers revealed their perception about healthy and nourished children, how to keep them healthy and the barriers on the way.

Mothers and grandmothers participated in the study. They mostly belong to scheduled caste family. Mother's age ranges from 17 to 25. Most of them are literate up to primary or secondary level.

They generally perceive under-nutrition is a state of health, not a disease. Regarding their child's health, they worry when their children fall ill with diarrhea or fever. Some of the caregivers in Krishnadaspur village perceive under-nutrition as a disease because doctors give vitamin tablets and syrups to cure under-nutrition. They also mentioned that their children are rural children so unless they refuse to eat, become very thin ("*khete chay na, roga hoye jay*") they presume that there is no need to give much attention to them as mothers of urban area do. "*sohorer bachhader moto oto ki gerame dekhasuno hoy*". In Krishnadaspur also, mothers perceive that children who less suffer from ailments, are not lazy, grow according to their age are healthy and nourished.

They understand that improper care during pregnancy increases the risk of childhood under-nutrition. Grandmother of one child under the age of three months argues that mother's proper care during pregnancy is responsible for child's nourishment. A mother of 1 and ½ year girl child agrees with the view and said that she thinks the cause of under-nutrition of her child lies in inadequate food intake by her during pregnancy. Now also they are unable to meet the food requirement everyday even for their children. Mothers in both the villages also reported that illness during pregnancy and related less food intake is also responsible for child's under-nutrition.

Younger mothers cannot make decisions about their children's feeding or care seeking. Only in laws and husband take decision about healthcare of children. Sometimes if husband remains busy with his work the family neglects the child's treatment. When the condition deteriorates then child is taken to the care provider. Such neglect is higher in case of elder children.

About child feeding different mothers have different opinions. Some of them believe in exclusive breastfeeding in adequate quantity whereas some others think babies need "Lactogen" (tined baby food) along with breast milk to remain healthy. Most of them believe that elder children need more calories so they must be given adequate vegetables, since fruit is costly. In Krishnadaspur, mothers said that due to less or no care during pregnancy some mothers have no or little breast milk and due to poor purchasing power they cannot provide other milk available in the market. So children become undernourished.

According to them, poor economic status and food insecurity serve inadequate meals to elder children. When they fall ill, do not get enough vegetables or fruits to meet the deficiency. Therefore they suffer frequently and such events increase the likelihood of under-nutrition among them. Mothers told that their children mostly suffer during summer. They also observed after suffering from ailments their children lose weight as evident from weight measurement in AWCs.

A Case Study

Sushama Saha, age 22 years, mother of two daughters – younger one is six months old – says that due to poor socioeconomic condition, her husband stays outside the state to earn more in order to nourish their children. So when her children fall ill, she is alone there to take them to doctor's clinic. Nobody is there to keep eye on the other child *e.g.* neighbor or family member. Though husband lives elsewhere he is the sole decision maker about their children and suggests treatment seeking. Only during emergency, neighbours ask about the incidence and suggest the treatment seeking. Husband sends money which is not sufficient to run the family. She had two cesarean operation so can't do heavy work. So it is difficult for her to provide proper care to her children. She says that when her duck lays egg, she try to sell it in the market instead of giving that egg for one day to one child (Author's work under SRTT fellowship in ISEC, Bangalore).

Mixed response came about the choice of provider; most of them prefer and visit qualified private provider in Rajrajeswarpur and RMP in Krishnadaspur. All of them in Rajrajeswarpur prefer treatment seeking from traditional healer for specific cases as well as when they do not see any improvement from allopathic medicines. *"onader daoa jolpora, nunpora ba telpora dile sarbei"*. But in Krishnadaspur, with increase in number of RMPs, reliance on traditional healers reduced (*"ekhon grame ekjon gunin ache tobe tar kachheo khub ekta keu jay na"*). Though some of them revealed their preference on 'gunin' when children behave unusually like cry longer, become senseless from time to time etc.

They generally provide homemade ORS during diarrhea since sometimes it becomes difficult to collect ORS and medicine from clinic at night. They mostly provide only ORS and no other food but some of them provide boiled semi solid food ("chira/rice"). AWW suggests about how to keep the child healthy. Mothers never ask the workers to weigh their child. They think AWW will weigh if they think it is necessary. Grandmothers have more observation power about symptomatic ailments. If any ailment requires hospitalization, they face problem with commute as boat is not available during night. So nearby doctor is the only resort. They get neighbour's help during treatment seeking to reach Sub Divisional Hospitals which are too far but they also have to bare food and lodging for them.

They all expressed that only home visit by AWW, provision of poor or average quality supplementary food or weighing of children are not sufficient to improve their children's health and nutritional status until and unless their socioeconomic condition improves and they become food secure, and if someone ensure availability of treatment and medicine even during night or climatic shock. *"kokhono kokhono sudhu alumulabhat juttechhe, kokhono ba tao jutchhe na, to kibhabe pustikor khabar khaoabo?"*

12

Econometric Model

This chapter includes econometric testing of the hypothesis through multivariate and bivariate logistic regression model. The econometric analysis (Table# 29) represents logistic regression models to explore whether different contextual factors increases the likelihood of under-nutrition significantly in the study area. Model 1 looks at the likelihood of association between household SES and stunting among children under the age of five in the two villages. Household's characteristics significantly increase the vulnerability to stunting in families who are more susceptible to chronic poverty according to poverty perception and lives in kutcha houses. Such factors become significant after controlling child specific factors. Living standard factor becomes insignificant after controlling of mother's perception and service delivery effectiveness and again becomes significant after controlling for impact of climatic shock on household SES. Vulnerability becomes higher among least poor families if impact of climatic shock is controlled.

Model 2 shows children of younger mothers; children of caregivers with good connection with health facility are more vulnerable to stunting. Mother's age becomes insignificant when child level factors, mother's perception and supply side environment are controlled. Earning member's workplace becomes significant after controlling the impact of climatic shock. It reflects that vulnerability to stunting is higher among children whose

Table# 29: The odds ratios from logistic regression to represent the influence of context on vulnerability to stunting

	Household characteristics	***Household and mother's characteristics***	***Household, mother and child's characteristics***	***Household, mother and child's characteristics with mother's perception and supply side***	***Previous model with interaction of climatic shock***
Moderate Poor	0.92	0.79	0.74	0.76	1.73
Least poor	0.89	1.04	1.02	0.96	123.23*
More vulnerable to chronic poverty	1.02	1.78	2.55*	2.39*	5.37
Semi-pucca house	0.39	0.32	.16*	0.17	.03***
20-25		0.52	0.65	0.64	1.29
26-30		.33*	0.43	0.44	0.50
30 & above		.29*	0.47	0.51	0.10
Have formal education		0.90	0.76	0.81	0.65
Father works outside the village		1.03	0.82	0.78	133.50*
Moderate connection with health facility		1.25	1.58	0.56	27.86*
Good connection with health facility		2.19**	2.14*	0.22	2.88
12-23			0.79	0.83	0.66
24-35			0.82	0.80	0.24
36 & above			.40*	.40*	0.22
Girl children			1.40	1.51	3.76**
Mother's perception about child health and nutritional status				.35*	
Mother's perception with moderate connection with health facility				2.16	

Table# 29: (*Contd...*)

Table# 29: (*Contd...*)

	House-hold chara-cteris-tics	***House-hold and mot-her's chara-cteris-tics***	***House-hold, mother and child's chara-cteris-tics***	***House-hold, mother and child's chara-cteris-tics with mother's percep-tion and supply side***	***Previous model with intera-ction of clim-atic shock***
Mother's perception with good connection with health facility				5.86**	
Climate impact index					4.12*
Moderate poor with moderate impact of climatic shock					0.50
Least poor with moderate to less impact of climatic shock					0.18
Working outside the village with moderate to less clim-atic impact					.089*
Number of observations	278	252	238	235	144
Wald chi^2	6.44	16.42	32.59	33.89	67.68
Prob>chi^2	0.7775	0.4943	0.1417	0.2045	0.0095
Pseudo R^2	0.0188	0.0597	0.1179	0.1371	0.3659

* p<.1; ** p<.05; *** p<.01

fathers work outside the village (within the GP, in different GP or in Kolkata) and also higher among children who have moderate connection with health facility. But in the final model it is evident that, the vulnerability to stunting becomes significantly higher for those children where earning members works inside village and face higher impact of climatic shock on house, land or other assets.

Younger children are more vulnerable to stunting which also remains significant even after controlling mother's perception and supply side effectiveness but becomes insignificant after controlling the impact of climatic shock. Vulnerability of girl children becomes significant after controlling of climatic shock impacts. Therefore, impact of climatic shock on SES increases the vulnerability to stunting for girl children irrespective of age significantly. Children are more vulnerable to stunting significantly if mothers perceive wrongly about their children's health and nutritional status even they have good contact and connections with health facilities.

The overall model becomes significant when interaction of climatic shock impact with SES, workplace, connection to health facility and feeding practice are incorporated. Keeping interaction of mother's perception with connection to supply side reduces the robustness of standard errors. So mother's perception is kept as a separate variable in the final model.

INFLUENCE OF DIFFERENT VULNERABILITIES ON CHILD'S AILMENT AND NUTRITIONAL STATUS

Prevalence of gastrointestinal problems in Krishnadaspur and Rajrajeswarpur are higher among medium vulnerable families as per climate impact index, least vulnerable in Krishnadaspur and medium vulnerable in Rajrajeswarpur as per livelihood insecurity index, among least vulnerable group according to physical inaccessibility index and higher among most vulnerable according to treatment seeking vulnerability index. With respect to stunting bivariate analyses depict that prevalence of stunting among children under the age of five is significantly higher among families who are most vulnerable according to impact of climatic shocks, livelihood insecurity, and physical inaccessibility in both the villages. But it is higher among least vulnerable families with respect to treatment seeking vulnerability index. Among the four models only the model livelihood insecurity is not significant overall. Results are evident from unadjusted odds ratios represented in the table below (Table# 30).

Table# 30: Unadjusted odds ratios to test the influence of contextual vulnerabilities on stunting in the study area

	Model treat-ment seeking	***Model climatic shock impact***	***Model liveli-hood in-security***	***Model physical inacces-sibility***
Treatment seeking vulnerability index				
Moderate vulnerable	0.82			
Less vulnerable	2.88**			
Climatic shock impact index				
Medium vulnerable		.47**		
Less vulnerable		.37***		
Livelihood insecurity index				
Moderately vulnerable livelihood			0.84	
Less vulnerable livelihood			.52*	
Physical inaccessibility index				
Moderate vulnerable physical accessibility				0.69
Less vulnerable physical accessibility				.38***
N	124	264	264	271
Wald chi^2	7.02	9.90	3.58	7.60
Prob>chi^2	0.0299	0.0071	0.1667	0.0223
Pseudo R^2	0.0522	0.0309	0.0121	0.0248

*p<.1; ** p<.05; *** p<.01

Conclusions

Thus it is evident from the above findings that multifaceted poverty is responsible for inequity in health seeking, differences in mother's knowledge, and practice regarding childcare. Such differential characteristics vary mostly between households within communities and less among communities. It is also evident that increased care with proper feeding of child at weaning period and universal health coverage for poor and backward social groups with proper family planning will help to reduce the prevalence. So bottom up strategies in policy development is to be strengthened through e-governance techniques along with effective and clear coordination among public health, nutrition and social departments to ensure universal access to public health goods and services along with effective communication strategy. India has much potential to address health equity through ongoing sectoral reforms. A common platform to approach health equity is to be built up to integrate departments, programmes, civil society organizations, researchers and ultimately vulnerable communities to accelerate the pace of inclusive growth and development.

Poor perception about child health and nutritional status, ineffective home visit of AWW, infrequent visits of them are more in non-deltaic village. Mother's poorly perceive about their children's health, and along with such perception most of them do not take their children to AWC everyday to receive supplementary nutrition. Even if they collect food for one child, share the same with one or two other members increasing the probability of undernourishment of the child. Most of them perceive that they are not insecure with supply of food during climatic shock episodes. But according to FGD, some of them argue that they really become insecure. In-depth interview with AWW reveals that though she suggests contingency plan to protect the child's care and feeding practice during climatic shock, mothers or caregivers do not feel the need and neglect the care even during normal time.

Thus non - deltaic village – less affected by impacts of climatic shock, less vulnerable with respect to livelihood insecurity, geographical adversity, accessibility to care provider – are more vulnerable to under-nutrition among children under the age of five with respect to supply side ineffectiveness compared to deltaic village. To improve child's nutritional status here, the effectiveness of ICDS centre should be modified according to area specific need. Some priority focus should be on –

1. Increase in the number of visits by AWW which should be done through strong monitoring system. It requires regular update of each child specific information in an electronic database
2. AWWs should record the advice digitally to keep record about the quality of need specific advices.
3. Digital recording of AWW level data monthly should comprise whether each and every child is visiting the centre everyday, whether they are eating the food in AWC, the amount of ration sanctioned per AWC and amount used everyday to prepare food per AWC, and quality of food should be checked with random visits.

Impact of climatic shock on infrastructures, assets, and livelihood is higher in deltaic village. But impact of service delivery is more or less same which shows massive ineffectiveness and negligence on the part of service delivery of health and nutrition. This leads to major dependence on rural unqualified provider in respect of care seeking and neglect on nutritional achievement since no private provider is there to watch, prevent and cure under-nutrition (one or two NGOs are working in some villages but not covering the whole).

Morbidity prevalence is higher among families who belong to poorest of the poor category, survives with subsistence level farming, fishing, honey or wood collection, livestock rearing or insignificant business and lives in poor environment. The evidence shows that mothers of some morbid children are literate up to primary level in deltaic village which indicates that firstly, education up to primary level is not sufficient to realize the need or degree of care giving and secondly impact of physical inaccessibility in this village is so strong that even mothers can feel the need, it is difficult for them to provide and increasing vulnerability to chronic poverty with time stops them to afford even lots of awareness generation campaigns take place. Limited level of understanding coupled with inaccessibility and lack of purchasing power acts as barrier to care seeking. Mother's early child bearing and related premature delivery increases the vulnerability of morbidity and under-nutrition among children more in deltaic village compared to non-deltaic village. Mother's under-nutrition influences under-nutrition more in non-deltaic village.

Though most of the mothers in Rajrajeswarpur perceive that their children are moderately healthy, most of the mothers of morbid children correctly perceive that their children are undernourished and suffer from ailments. Even though they are literate or educated up to primary level, they do not follow proper feeding practice *e.g.*, continuation of breastfeeding along with complementary feeding during weaning period due to poor community level services delivered by ICDS centre.

In both the villages, prevalence of stunting is influenced by climatic, geographic and socioeconomic vulnerabilities. Among those, vulnerable impact of climatic shock is the most significant one. In other words, stunting prevalence is higher among children who live in most vulnerable area according to climatic shock proneness.

In non-deltaic village, the most significant vulnerability is ineffective service delivery comprising non-availability of medicine, overcrowding of health centres, preference of home delivery with help of dai or RMP, higher charge of RMPs during climatic shocks, relying on RMPs for care seeking. Children who are under 5 months of age, smaller at birth and girl children are more stunted strengthens the argument regarding the existence of intergenerational transfer of under-nutrition and gender discrimination in deltaic village– another dimension of social vulnerability. Social acceptability of health seeking to unqualified provider is more in non-deltaic village where most of the households perceive that institutional delivery or care seeking from qualified provider is costly compared to home delivery or care seeking from RMP, and also family tradition prohibits to seek care from institution. With respect to healthcare expenditure, Krishnadaspur is more vulnerable to chronic poverty due to expenditure on medicine and Rajrajeswarpur becomes vulnerable due to higher doctor fees.

In respect of community responsiveness to help treatment seeking during normal time or in emergency, though villagers get moderate help from their neighbours, limited or very little attention is received from NGOs or CBOs.

In both the villages, morbidity and under-nutrition prevalence is higher among families perceiving that the pattern of movement in economic status was not so alarming. But as per perception about current socioeconomic status, most poor with severe economic status fall shares higher burden of under-nutrition in deltaic village and higher toll of morbidity in non-deltaic village. Most of the families having morbid or undernourished children in deltaic village do not perceive that impact of health expenditure is higher during climatic shock and due to that economic status deterioration are moderate or high which is just opposite in non-deltaic village. But mothers of undernourished children in both the villages compared to mothers of morbid children have wrong perception about food insecurity even they do food consumption sacrifice (more than 75 percent families) after health expenditure.

Though inhabitants suffer a lot, they are not ready to migrate due to poor economic status. Most of them works in agricultural land, do fishing or work in other's house as each and every work is seasonal in nature. So, uncertain livelihood will become more uncertain if they move to new place. They all agree about the fact that socioeconomic status, uncertain livelihood, societal system, governance and administration, health and nutrition service delivery – all are linked with child health and nutritional status. However, they want more stress on improvement on economic status through stable livelihood and child health above all. Few policy suggestions will be -

- Generate the scope of work through making the site more attractive for tourists
- Scientific way for reducing salinity
- Regulating food and healthcare market through
    - Price ceiling of major food crops and monitoring it effectively
    - Make the essential medicines easily available
    - Provide training to RMPs and monitor them on regular basis to minimize the risk
    - Quality and effectiveness measure of ICDS and healthcare provider in fixed interval
    - Strengthening monitoring of ICDS centres
- Creating more involvement of community through active cooperation of SHGs.

Actual economic status fall due to health expenditure, limited purchasing power due to chronic poverty causing limited access to food, limited availability of food in the market due to lack of production as a consequence of climatic shock induced productivity loss, high price due to shortage of supply – leads to lack of effective demand for food in both the deltaic and non-deltaic village. All these coupled with wrong perception about food insecurity, about subjective economic status fall even after consumption sacrifice, limits the demand for food among families of undernourished children in deltaic village. But in non-deltaic village, even there is perception of subjective economic status fall, wrong perception about food insecurity limits the demand among families of undernourished children. In addition to this, physical inaccessibility to care providers in deltaic village even with moderate effectiveness of health and nutrition service delivery, higher cost of medicines and doctor fees leading to improper treatment seeking from traditional healers or relying on home remedies in both the villages and ineffective service delivery leading to poor childcare and feeding in non-deltaic village contributes to morbidity and under-nutrition. Therefore social adaptation against no or little economic resilience, little community involvement leads to sub-optimal solutions to health and nutritional status and limited ability to adapt against socioeconomic, livelihood related vulnerabilities coupled with climatic shocks reduces the capacity to combat under-nutrition. Therefore under-nutrition-morbidity vicious circle is very common scenario in such context leading to chronic under-nutrition given the context[1].

[1] Bibliography will be available upon request

References

Abeykoon A.T. (1995). "Sex preference in South Asia: Sri Lanka an outlier." *Asia-Pacific Population Journal*, 10(3): 5-16.

ACC/SCN. (1997). "Nutrition and Poverty". Papers from the SCN 24th Session Symposium in Kathmandu. *ACC/SCN Symposium Report*, Nutrition Policy.

Alderman H., Hoddinott J., Kinsey B. (2006). "Long term consequences of early childhood malnutrition", *Oxford Economic Papers*, Oxford University Press. 58(3): 450-474.

Alwang J., Siegel P.B., Jorgensen, S.L. (2001) "Vulnerability: A View from Different Disciplines". *Social Protection Discussion Paper Series*, The World Bank, Washington DC.

Andersen R.M., and Davidson P.L. (2001). "Improving access to care in America: Individual and contextual indicators. In Changing the U.S. health care system: Key issues in health services, policy and management", edited by R. Andersen, T. Rice, and J. Kominski, 3-30. San Francisco: Jossey-Bass.

Andersen R.M. (1995). "Revisiting the behavioural model and access to medical care: Does it matter?" *Journal of Health & Social Behaviour*, 36(1), 1-10.

Anderson R.M. (2008). "National health surveys and the behavioral model of health services use", *Medical Care*, 46(7): 647-53.

Anoop, S., Saravanan, B., Joseph, A., Cherian, A., Jacob, K.S. (2004). "Maternal depression and low maternal intelligence as risk factors for malnutrition in children: a community based case-control study from South India", *Archives of Disease in Childhood*, 89(4): 325-329.

Arnold, F., Nangia, P., Kapil, U. (2004). "Indicators of nutrition for women and children: current status and recommendations", *Economic and Political Weekly*, 39(7): 664-670.

Asian Development Bank. (2001). "Social Protection in Asia and the Pacific". Asian Development Bank, Manila.

Aturupane, H., Deolalikar, A., Gunewardena, D. (2008). *The Determinants of Child Weight and Height in Sri Lanka: A Quantile Regression Approach*, UNU-WIDER Research Paper No. 2008/53, World Institute of Development Economic Research, Helsinki.

References

Ayeni B., Rushton G., McNulty M.L. (1987). "Improving the geographical accessibility of health care in rural areas: a Nigerian case study." *Social Science & Medicine* 25(10): 1083-1094.

Azam S. and Imai K.S. (2009). "Vulnerability and Poverty in Bangladesh". Chronic Poverty Research Centre, University of Manchester, UK.

Baeza C. and Packard T. (2006). "Beyond Survival Protecting Households from Health Shocks in Latin America". The World Bank, Washington DC. http://dx.doi.org/10.1596/978-0-8213-6571-7

Bairagi R. (1986). "Food crisis, nutrition, and female children in rural Bangladesh." *Population and Development Review,* 307-315.

Bamji M.S. (2003). "Early nutrition and health-Indian perspective", *Current Science*, 85: 1137–1142.

Barrera A. (1990). "The role of maternal schooling and its interaction with public health programs in child health production". *Journal of Development Economics*, 32(1): 69-91.

Basta, S.S., Darwin K., Scrimshaw N.S. (1979). "Iron deficiency anemia and the productivity of adult males in Indonesia." *American Journal of Clinical Nutrition,* 32(4): 916-25.

Bawdekar M., Singh L.L. (2008). "Contextual correlates of child malnutrition in rural Maharashtra", *Journal of Biosocial Science*, 40: 771-786.

Bebbington A. (1999). "Capitals and Capabilities: A Framework for Analyzing Peasant Viability, Rural Livelihoods and Poverty". *World Development*, 27: 2021-2034.

Begum S., Sen B. (2004). "Unsustainable livelihoods, health shocks and urban chronic poverty: rickshaw pullers as a case study."

Behrman J.R., Deolalikar A.B. (1988). "Health and Nutrition", in Hollis Chenery & T.N. Srinivasan (eds.), *Handbook on Economic Development*, Elsevier, 1(14): 631-711.

Bentley M.E. (1988). "The Household Management of Childhood Diarrhea in Rural North India." *Social Science & Medicine*, 27:75-85. http://dx.doi.org/10.1016/0277-9536(88)90165-7

Bharati S., Pal M., Bharati P. (2008). "Determinants of nutritional status of pre-school children in India", *Journal of Biosocial Science*, 40: 801-814.

Bingenheimer, J.B., Raudenbush., S.W. (2004). "Statistical and substantive inferences in public health: issues in the application of multilevel models". *Annual Review of Public Health*, 25: 53-77.

Black R.E., Mathers, C., Rivera J., Caulfield L.E., Allen L.H., Ezzati M., Onis M., Bhutta Z.A. (2008). "Maternal and child under-nutrition: Global and regional exposures and health consequences". *Lancet Series: Maternal and Child Under-nutrition 1*, 371(9608), 243-60.

Blackie, P., Cannon, T., Davis, I. and Wisner, B. (1994). "At Risk: Natural Hazards, People's Vulnerability and Disasters". Routledge, New York.

Bradley, R.H., and Corwyn R.F. (2002). "Socioeconomic status and child development." *Annual Review of Psychology* 53(1): 371-399.

Braveman, P. (2006). "Health disparities and health equity: concepts and measurement", Annual *Review of Public Health*, 27: 167-194.

Brennan, L., McDonald, J., Shlomowitz, R. (2004). "Infant feeding practices and chronic child malnutrition in the Indian state of Karnataka and Uttar Pradesh", *Economics and Human Biology*, 2(1): 139-158.

Briend A., Wojtyniak B., Rowland M.G.M. (1988). "Breast feeding, nutritional state, and child survival in rural Bangladesh." *British medical journal* (Clinical research ed.) 296(6626): 879.

Brockerhoff M., Hewett P. (2000). "Inequality of child mortality among ethnic groups in sub-Saharan Africa." *Bulletin of the World Health Organization*, 78(1): 30-41.

Budowski M., Bixby L.R. (2003). "Fatherless Costa Rica: Child acknowledgment and support among lone mothers." *Journal of Comparative Family Studies,*: 229-254.

Bureau, Washington DC.

Caldwell J.C. (1979). "Education as a Factor in Mortality Decline An Examination of Nigerian Data". *Population Studies*. 33(3): 395-413.

Caldwell, J.C. (1993). "Health transition: The cultural, social and behavioural determinants of health in the third World". *Social Science & Medicine*, 36(2): 125-135.

Calvo C., S. Dercon. (2005). "Measuring individual vulnerability". Economics Series Working Paper No. 229. Department of Economics, University of Oxford, Oxford.

Carr, D. (2004). "Improving the Health of the World's poorest people", *Health Bulletin*. In Vol. 1. Population Reference.

Caulfield L.E., Onis M., Blossner M., Black R.E. 2004. Undernutrition as an underlying cause of child deaths associated with diarrhea, pneumonia, malaria, and measles. *American Journal of Clinical Nutrition*. Vol. 80: pp: 193–198.

Census (2011) Government of India.

Chakrabarty, A. (2004). "Determinants of Child Morbidity and Factors Governing Utilization of Child Health Care: Evidence from Rural India", *Working Paper*. Jawaharlal Nehru University – CESP, New Delhi.

Chambers R. (1989) "Vulnerability, Coping and Policy". Editorial Introduction, *IDS Bulletin*, 20, 1-7. http://dx.doi.org/10.1111/j.1759-5436.1989.mp20002001.x

Chhotray V., Roger F. (2012). "Post-disaster recovery and ongoing vulnerability: Ten years after the super-cyclone of 1999 in Orissa, India." *Global Environmental Change* 22(3): 695-702.

Claeson M., Bos E.R., Mawji T. (2000). "Reducing child mortality in India in the new millennium", *Bulletin of World Health Organization*, 78(10): 1192-1199.

Coudouel A., Hentschel J. (2000). "Poverty Data and Measurement". Preliminary Draft for a Sourcebook on Poverty Reduction Strategies. The World Bank, Washington DC.

Cutter S.L., Boruff B.J., Shirley W.L. (2003). "Social vulnerability to environmental hazards", *Social Science Quarterly*, 84(2), 242-61.

Dasgupta P., Ray, D. (1986). "Inequality as a Determinant of Malnutrition and Unemployment: Theory", *The Economic Journal*, 96(384): 1011-1034.

Dasgupta P., Ray, D. (1987). "Inequality as a determinant of malnutrition and unemployment: policy." *The Economic Journal*, 97(385): 177-188.

Daulaire N.M., *et al.* "Childhood mortality after a high dose of vitamin A in a high risk population." *British Medical Journal*, 304(6821): 207-210.

Deolalikar A. (2004). "Poverty and Child Malnutrition in Bangladesh". The World Bank, Washington DC.

Dercon S. (2005). "Risk, vulnerability and poverty in Africa." *Journal of African Economies*.

Dercon, S. (2011). "Social Protection, Efficiency and Growth". CSAE Working Paper WPS/2011-17, Oxford University, Oxford.

Devereux G., Turner S.W., Craig L.C., McNeill G., Martindale S., Harbour P.J., Seaton A. (2006). "Low maternal vitamin E intake during pregnancy is associated with asthma in 5-year-old children". *American Journal of Respiratory and Critical Care Medicine*, 174(5), 499-507.

Dutta A., Pant K. (2003). "The nutritional status of indigenous people in the Garhwal Himalayas, India." *Mountain Research and Development* 23(3): 278-283.

Elfindri (1993). Nutritional status of elementary school aged children in a rural population. *Indonesian Journal of Demography* 20: 31-49.

Ellbers C. and Gunning J. (2003) Growth and Risk: Methodology and Micro-Evidence. Tinbergen Institute Discussion Papers, 03-068/2.

Enarson E. (2000). Gender equality, work and disaster reduction: Making the connections. Presented at the ILO in Focus Programme on Crisis Response and Reconstruction.

Esrey S.A., *et al.* (1988). "Drinking water source, diarrheal morbidity, and child growth in villages with both traditional and improved water supplies in rural Lesotho, southern Africa." *American Journal of Public Health,* 78(11): 1451-1455.

Fajth. (2009). "Joint Statement on Child Sensitive Social Protection". Presentation at Social Protection Floor Initiative, Turin.

Fotso J.C. (2006) "Child Health Inequities in Developing Countries: Differences across Urban and Rural Areas". *International Journal for Equity in Health,* 5(9), http://dx.doi.org/10.1186/1475-9276-5-9

Fotso J.C., Firestone R. (2008). Maternal education or household wealth: Which is the best predictor of child malnutrition in Sub-Saharan Africa? Population Association of America Annual Meeting Programme, USA.

Fotso J.C., Kuate-Defo B. (2006). "Household and community socioeconomic influences on early childhood malnutrition in Africa", *Journal of Biosocial Science*, 38(3): 289-313.

Galobardes, Bruna, John W. Lynch, and George Davey Smith. (2004). "Childhood socioeconomic circumstances and cause-specific mortality in adulthood: systematic review and interpretation." *Epidemiologic Reviews,* 26(1): 7-21.

Garcia M. (1994). Malnutrition and food insecurity projections2020, 2020 Brief no. 6, International Food Policy Research Institute, Washington, DC.

Garrett J.L. (2000). Achieving urban food and nutrition security in the developing world. Overview. A 2020 vision for food, agriculture and the environment. *Focus* 3. (Brief 1 of 10), International Food Policy Research Institute, Washington, DC.

Ghosh R. (2012). "Child mortality in India: a complex situation", *World Journal of Pediatrics*, 8(1): 11-18.

Ghosh S., Shah D. (2004). "Nutritional problems in urban slum children". *Indian Pediatrics*, 41(7): 682-696.

Giashuddin M.S., Kabir M. Hasan M. (2005) "Economic Disparity and Child Nutrition in Bangladesh". *Indian Journal of Pediatrics*, 72, 481-487. http://dx.doi.org/10.1007/BF02724424

Gilson L., McIntyre D. (2001). "South Africa: Addressing the legacy of apartheid". In Evans, T., Whitehead, M., Diderichsen, F., Bhuiya, A. and Wirth, M. (*eds*), Challenging Inequities in Health: From Ethics to Action. Oxford University Press, New York, pp. 190-209.

Gopalan S.S., Mohanty S., Das A. (2011). "Challenges and opportunities for policy decisions to address health equity in developing health systems: case study of the policy processes in the Indian state of Orissa", *International Journal for Equity in Health*, 10:55.

Gragnolati M., Shekar M., Das Gupta M., Bredenkamp C., Lee Y.K. (2005). "India's undernourished children: a call for reform and action", *Health, Nutrition and Population Discussion Paper*, The World Bank, Washington DC.

Gragnolati, M. (1999). "Children's Growth and Poverty in Rural Guatemala", *World Bank Policy Research Working Paper No. 2193.* The World Bank, Washington DC.

Gregory P.J., Ingram J.S., Brklacich M. (2005). Climate change and food security. *Philosophical Transactions of the Royal Society B* 360, 2139–48.

Grossman, Michael. (1972). "The demand for health: a theoretical and empirical investigation." National Bureau of Economic Research, ISBN - 0-87014-248-8

Gupta N., Zurn P., Diallo K., Poz. M.R.D. (2003). "Uses of population census data for monitoring geographical imbalance in the health workforce: snapshots from three developing countries", *International Journal of Equity in Health,* 2(11).

Gwatkin D.R., Ruston S., Johnson K., Paned R.P., Wagstaff A. (2000). "Socioeconomic differences in health, nutrition and population in

Bangladesh", *Health, Nutrition and Population Discussion Paper*, The World Bank, Washington DC.

Gwatkin D.R., Bhuiya A., Victora C.G. (2004). "Making health systems more equitable", *The Lancet*, 364(9441): 1273-1280.

Gwatkin D.R., Rutstein S., Johnson K., Suliman E., Wagstaff A., Amouzou A. (2007). "Socio-economic differences in health, nutrition, and population within developing countries. An overview", *Country report on HNP and Poverty*, The World Bank, Washington DC.

Haddad L., Alderman H., Appleton S., Song L., Yohannes Y. (2003). Reducing child malnutrition: How far does income growth take us? *The World Bank Economic Review*, 17(1), 107-131.

Haddad L., Bhattarai S., Immink M. Kumar S. (1995). "Household food security and diarrhoea as determinants of nutrition: New trade-offs and new opportunities towards 2020?" *Discussion Paper*, International Food Policy Research Institute, Washington, DC.

Harttgen K., Misselhorn M. (2006). A multilevel approach to explain child mortality and under-nutrition in South Asia and Sub-Saharan Africa, *Discussion Papers 152*, America Institute for Economic Research, Great Barrington, MA.

Heady P., Kohli M. (2010). "Introduction: Towards a political economy of kinship and welfare." Family, kinship and state in contemporary Europe: Vol. 3; Perspectives on Theory and Policy. 15-30.

Heller P., Drake W. (1979). "Malnutrition, child morbidity, and the family decision process". *Journal of Development Economics,* 6(21): 203-35.

Heltberg R. (2009). "Malnutrition, poverty and economic growth". *Economics of Health and Social Care*, 18(S1): S77-S88.

Heuveline P., Goldman N. (2000). "A description of child illness and treatment behavior in Guatemala". *Social Science and Medicine*, 50(3): 345-364.

Hewett P.C., Montgomery M.R. (2001). "Poverty and public services in developing-country cities". *Policy Research Division Working Paper* 154. The Population Council.

Himanshu H., Stern N. (2011). "India and an Indian village: 50 years of economic development in Palanpur". Working Paper, 43. Asia Research Centre, London School of Economics and Political Science, London, UK.

Holzmann R., Jorgensen S. (1999). "Social Protection as Social Risk Management: Conceptual Underpinnings for the Social Protection Sector Strategy Paper". The World Bank, Washington DC.

Hong R., Banta J., Betancourt J. (2006). "Relationship between household wealth inequality and chronic childhood under-nutrition in Bangladesh", *International Journal for Equity in Health*, 5:15.

Hong R., Mishra V. (2006). "Effect of Wealth Inequality on Chronic Under-Nutrition in Cambodian Children". *Journal of Health and Population Nutrition*, 24, 89-99.

Houweling T.A., Ronsmans C., Campbell M.R.O., Kunst A.E. (2007). "Huge poor-rich inequalities in maternity and child care in developing countries", *Bulletin of the World Health Organization*, 85(10): 745-754. http://www.who.int/globalchange/news/fsclimandhealth/en/

http://dx.doi.org/10.1016/S0305-750X(99)00104-7

IIPS (International Institute of Population Sciences and ORC Macro) (2007). National Family Health Survey Report.

Imai K.S., Annim S.K., Kulkarni V.S., Gaiha R. (2014). Women's empowerment and prevalence of stunted and underweight children in Rural India. *World Development*, 62, 88-105.

Immink M. DC., Viteri F. E. (1981). "Energy intake and productivity of Guatemalan sugarcane cutters: An empirical test of the efficiency wage hypothesis part I." *Journal of Development Economics* 9(2): 251-271.

Immink, M. DC, and Viteri F. E. (1981). "Energy intake and productivity of Guatemalan sugarcane cutters: An empirical test of the efficiency wage hypothesis part II." *Journal of Development Economics*, 9(2): 273-287.

Indian Council of Medical Research. (1972). *Growth and Physical Development of Indian Infants and Children*, Technical Report, Vol. 18, India.

Indian Council of Medical Research. 2003. Health status of primitive tribes of Orissa. ICMR Bulletin. 33(10): 1-8.

Institute of Health Management Research (2010) Health Care in the Sundarbans (India): Challenges and Plan for a Better Future. www.futurehealthsystems.org

International Institute for Population Sciences (IIPS) & ORC MACRO. 2000. National Family Health Survey (NFHS-II), 1998-99, Mumbai, India.

International Institute for Population Sciences (IIPS) & ORC MACRO. 1994. National Family Health Survey (NFHS-I) 1992-93, Mumbai, India.

Jayachandran S., Pande R. (2012). "The Puzzle of High Child Malnutrition in South Asia." presentation slides, International Growth Centre, London School of Economics, UK.

Jonathan K., Dorward A., Poulton C. (2002). "Institutional dimensions of trade liberalisation and poverty". Paris, France. www.sarpn.org/wssd/agriculture/kydd/Trade.pdf

Jones A. P., Bentham G., Horwell C. (1999). "Health service accessibility and deaths from asthma." *International Journal of Epidemiology*, 28(1): 101-105.

Jordan H., Roderick P., Martin D., Barnett S. (2004). "Distance, rurality and the need for care: access to health services in South West England", *International Journal of Health Geographics*, 3: 21.

Kanjilal B., Mazumdar P.G., Mukherjee M., Rahamn M.H. (2010). "Nutritional status of children in India: household socio-economic condition as the contextual determinant", *International Journal for Equity in Health*, 9:19.

Kanjilal B., Mukherjee M., Singh S., Mondal S., Barman D., Mandal A. (2007). Health, Equity and Poverty Exploring the Links in West Bengal, India, *Future Health Systems Working paper 4*. India series, West Bengal. www.futurehealthsystems.org.

Kapur D., Sharma S., Agarwal K.N. (2005). "Dietary intake and growth pattern of children 9-36 months of age in an urban slum in Delhi'. *Indian Pediatrics*. Vol. 42.

Larrea C., Freire W. (2002). Social Inequality and Child Malnutrition in Four Andean Countries. *Revista Panamericana de Salud Pública, 11, 356-364. http://dx.doi.org/10.1590/S1020-49892002000500010*

Larrea, C., Kawachi I. (2005). "Does economic inequality affect child malnutrition? The case of Ecuador", *Social Science & Medicine*, 60(1): 165-178.

Lawn J.E., Tinker A., Mridha M.K., Anwar I. (2006). "Where is maternal and child health now?" *The Lancet*, 368(9546): 1474-1477.

Leibenstein H. (1957). "The theory of underemployment in backward economies." *Journal of Political Economy,* 65(2): 91-103.

Ligon E. Schechter L. (2003) Measuring Vulnerability. *The Economic Journal*, 113, C95-C102. http://dx.doi.org/10.1111/1468-0297.00117

Linnemayr S., Ka A., Alderman H. (2008). "Determinants of malnutrition in Senegal: Individual, household, community variables, and their interaction". *Economics & Human Biology*, 6(2): 252–63.

Lutter C.K., Mora J.O., Habicht J.P., Rasmussen K.M., Robson D.S., Sellers S.G., Herrera M.G. (1989). Nutritional supplementation: effects on child stunting because of diarrhea. *The American Journal of Clinical Nutrition*, 50(1): 1-8.

Magadi M. (2004). "Maternal and Child Health among the Urban Poor in Nairobi, Kenya". *African Population Studies*, 19.

Mahal A., Yazbeck A.S., Peters D.H., Ramana G.N.V. (2001). "The poor and health service use in India". *Health, Nutrition and Population Discussion Paper*, The World Bank, Washington DC.

Mamobolo R., Alberts M., Steyn N.P., Delemarre-van de Waal H.A., Levitt N.S. (2005). "Prevalence and determinants of stunting and overweight in 3-year-old black South African children residing in the Central Region of Limpopo Province, South Africa", *Public Health Nutrition*, 8(5): 501–508.

Mani S. (2007). The Role of the Household and Community in Determining Child Health, *UNU-WIDER Research Paper No. 2007/78*, Helsinki, Finland.

Marini A., Gragnolati M. (2006). "Non-linear effects of Altitude on Child growth in Peru: A Multilevel Analysis". *World Bank Policy research Working Paper* No. 3823.The World Bank, Washington DC.

Marta M.J., Carr D.L., Funk C., Husak G.J., Chafe Z.A. (2012). "Climate change and human health: Spatial modeling of water availability, malnutrition, and livelihoods in Mali, Africa". *Applied Geography*, 33: 4-15.

Martorell R., Ho T.J. (1984). "Under-nutrition, morbidity and mortality", *Population and development review*, supplement to Vol. 10: in Mosley, H. and Chen, L.C. (eds), Child Survival: Strategies for Research, Cambridge University Press, Cambridge, pp. 49-68.

Maxwell D., Levin C., Armar-Klemesu M., Ruel M., Morris S., Ahaideke C. (2000). "Urban Livelihoods and Food and Nutrition Security in Greater Accra, Ghana". *Research Report 112*, International Food Policy Research Institute (IFPI), Washington DC.

Menon P., Ruel M.T., Morris S.S. (2000). "Socio-economic differentials in child stunting are consistently larger in urban than in rural areas", *Food and Nutrition Bulletin*, 21(3): 282–289.

Mertens J., *et al.* (1990). "On predatory tendencies in the feeding ecology of the fairy shrimp Streptocephalus proboscideus (Frauenfeld, 1873) (Crustacea: Anostraca)." Intrazooplankton Predation. Springer Netherlands, 119-123.

Mishra V.K., Rutherford R.D. (2000). "Women's Education Can Improve Child Nutrition in India", *NFHS Bulletin*. Vol. 15.

Mohanty S.K., Pathak P.K. (2009). "Rich-poor gap in utilization of reproductive and child health services in India, 1992-2005", *Journal of Biosocial Science*, 41(3): 381-398.

Monteiro C., D'Aquino Benicio M.H., Conde W.L., Konno S., Lovadino A.L., Barros A.J.D., Victora C.G. (2009). "Narrowing socioeconomic inequality in child stunting: The Brazilian experience (1974-2007)", *Bulletin of the World Health Organization*, 88(4): 305-311.

Montgomery M.R. (2009). "Urban Poverty and Health in Developing Countries. *Population Bulletin*". 64 (2).

Montgomery M.R., Hewett P.C. (2005). "Urban poverty and health in developing countries: Household and neighbourhood effects", *Demography*, 42(3): 397-425.

Montgomery Mark R., *et al.* (2001). "Social networks and contraceptive dynamics in Southern Ghana." *Policy Research Division Working Paper* 153.

Morales R., A.M. Aguilar, & A. Calzadilla (2004). Geography and culture matter for malnutrition in Bolivia. *Economics & Human Biology*, 2(3), 373–89.

Morris S.S. (2000). Targeting urban malnutrition: A multicity analysis of the spatial distribution of childhood nutritional status, *FCND Discussion Paper No. 94*, International Food Policy Research Institute, Washington, DC.

Morrow B.H. (1999). "Identifying and mapping community vulnerability". *Disasters* 24, 1–18.

Moser S.C., and Ekstrom. J.A. (2010). "A framework to diagnose barriers to climate change adaptation." *Proceedings of the National Academy of Sciences* 107.51: 22026-22031.

Moser, C. and Holland, J. (1997) Household Responses to Poverty and Vulnerability, Volume 4: Confronting Crisis in Cawama, Lusaka, Zambia.

Urban Management Programme Policy Paper, UMPP No. 24. The World Bank, Washington DC. http://dx.doi.org/10.1596/0-8213-3850-1

Mosley W.H., Chen L.C. (1984). An analytical framework for the study of child survival in developing countries. *Population and Development Review* 10 (Supplement), 25–45.

Mukherjee M.(2014). Ex Ante Inequality and Under-Nutrition Vulnerability Dynamics: Case Study of the Sundarbans Delta Region, West Bengal, India. Food and Nutrition Sciences, 2014, 5, 1951-1963. http://dx.doi.org/10.4236/fns.2014.520207

Mukherjee M., Kanjilal B., Barman D., Mazumdar P.G. (2012) Child Health in the Sundarbans: How Far Mutually Reinforcing Shocks Act as Contextual Determinants? *Journal of Health Management*, 14: 117-140. http://dx.doi.org/10.1177/097206341201400203

Naidoo J. (2009). "Food for thought at Copenhagen". *The Hindu*, 7 December. Available at http://beta.thehindu. com/opinion/op-ed/article61098.ece

Navaneetham K., Jose S. (2005). "Poverty, malnutrition and mortality in south Asia: A review of issues and options". Trivandrum: Centre for Development Studies.

O'Donnell O., Van Doorslaer E., Wagstaff A., Lindelow M. (2008) "Analyzing Health Equity Using Household Survey Data". The World Bank, Washington DC.

Omitsu M. Yamano T. (2006). "The impacts of hurricane mitch on child health: Evidence from Nicaragua". Presented at the International Association of Agricultural Economists Conference, Gold Coast, Australia.

Onis M., Frongillo E.A., Blossner M. (2000). "Is malnutrition declining? An analysis of changes in levels of child malnutrition since 1980", *Bulletin of the World Health Organization*. 78: 1222–1233.

Oomann N., Lule E., Chhabra R. (2003). "Inequalities in health, nutrition and population- Rajasthan, India". *Health, Nutrition and Population Discussion Paper*, The World Bank, Washington DC.

Oppong J.R., Hodgson M.J. (2005). "Spatial Accessibility to Health care facilities in Suhum District, Ghana". *The Professonal Geographer*, 46(2):1999-209

Padmadas S.S., Hutter I., Willekens F. (2002). "Weaning initiation patterns and subsequent linear growth progression among children aged 2-4 years in India", *International Journal of Epidemiology*, 31(4): 855-863.

Pal, S. (1999). "An analysis of childhood malnutrition in rural India: Role of gender, income and other household characteristics", *World Development*, 27(7): 1151–1171.

Pathak P.K., Singh A. (2009). "Geographical variation in poverty and child malnutrition in India" in Singh, K.K., Yadava, R.C., Pandey, A. (eds), *Population, poverty and health: analytical approaches*, Hindustan Publishing Corporation, New Delhi, India, pp. 183-206.

Pebley A.R., Amin S. (1991). "The impact of public health interventions on sex differentials in childhood mortality in rural Punjab India."

Pelletier D.L. (1994). "The relationship between child anthropometry and mortality in developing countries: implications for policy, programs and future research." *The Journal of nutrition,* 124(10): 2047S.

Perry B. Gesler W. (2000). "Physical access to primary health care in Andean Bolivia." *Social Science & Medicine* 50.9: 1177-1188.

Peters D.H., Garg A., Walker D.G., Bloom G., Rahman M.H., Brieger W.R. (2008). "Poverty and access to healthcare in developing countries". *Annals of the New York Academy of Science*, 1136, 161–71.

Planning Commission, Government of India. 2001. National Human Development Report.

Poel E., Hosseinpoor A., Appiah C., Vega J., Speybroeck N. (2007). "Malnutrition and the disproportional burden on the poor: The case of Ghana." *International Journal for Equity in Health*, 6(21), 1–12.

Poel E., Hosseinpoor A., Speybroeck N., Ourti T., Vega J. (2008) "Socioeconomic Inequality in Malnutrition in Developing Countries". *Bulletin of the World Health Organization*, 86, 282-291. http://dx.doi.org/10.2471/BLT.07.044800

Pongou R., Ezzati M., Salomon J.A. (2006). "Household and Community Socioeconomic and Environmental Determinants of Child Nutritional Status in Cameroon". *BMC Public Health*, 6, 98. http://dx.doi.org/10.1186/1471-2458-6-98

Radhakrishna R., Rao K.H., Ravi C., Reddy B.S. (2006). "Estimation and Determination of Chronic Poverty in India: An Alternative Approach". Paper presented at the CPRC Workshop on 'Concepts and Methods for Analysing Poverty Dynamics and Chronic Poverty', Chancellors Conferencc Center, University of Manchester.

Radhakrishna R., Ravi C. (2004)."Malnutrition in India. Economic and Political Weekly", 39: 671–676.

Rahman S., Smith D.K. (2000). "Use of location-allocation models in health service development planning in developing nations". *European Journal of Operational Research*, 53(3):437-452

Rahmathullah L. et al. (1990). "Reduced mortality among children in southern India receiving a small weekly dose of vitamin A." *New England Journal of Medicine,* 323(14): 929-935.

Raj, A., McDougal, L.P. & Silverman, J.G. (2015). "Gendered Effects of Siblings on Child Malnutrition in South Asia: Cross-sectional Analysis of Demographic and Health Surveys from Bangladesh, India, and Nepal", *Maternal Child Health Journal*, 19: 217

Rajaram S., Sunil T.S., Zottarelli L.K. (2003). "An analysis of childhood malnutrition in Kerala and Goa", *Journal of Biosocial Science*. 35(3): 335-351.

Rajaram S., Zottarelli L.K., Sunil T.S. (2007). "Individual, household, programme and community effects on childhood malnutrition in rural India", *Maternal and Child Nutrition*, 3(2): 129-140.

Ramalingaswami V., Johnsson U., Rohde J. (1996). "The Asian Enigma. Progress of Nations", United Nations Children's Fund.

Rao D.H., Rao M.K. (1994). "Levels of malnutrition and socio-economic conditions among Maria Gonds", *Journal of Human Ecology*, 5: 185–190.

Rao G.R., Singh L.L., Pritamjit R. (2004). "Nutritional status of children in Northeast India", *Asia Pacific Population Journal*, 19: 39–56.

Ravallion M. (1998). "Poverty Lines in Theory and Practice". *Living Standards Measurement Study, Working Paper No.133*, World Bank, Washington DC.

Reardon T., Vosti S. (1995). "Links between Rural Poverty and the Environment in Developing Countries: Asset Categories and Investment Poverty". *World Development*, 23, 1495-1506. http://dx.doi.org/10.1016/0305-750X(95)00061-G.

Reed *et al.* 2010

Rice N., Jones A. (1997): "Multi level Models and Health Economics". *Health Economics*. 6(6): 561-575.

Roetten K., Sabates-Wheeler R. (2011). "A Child Sensitive Approach to Social Protection: Serving Practical and Strategic Needs." *Proceedings of the Conference "Social Protection for Social Justice"*, London, 13-15 April 2011.

Rosenzweig M.R., Schultz T.P. (1982). "Child mortality and fertility in Colombia: Individual and community effects". *Health Policy and Education*, 2(3–4): 305–48.

Ruel M.T. (2000). "Urbanization in Latin America: Constraints and opportunities for child feeding and care". *Food and Nutrition Bulletin*, 21(1): 12–24.

Ruel M.T., Garrett J.L. (2004). "Features of urban food and nutrition security and consideration for successful urban programming". *Electronic Journal of Agriculture and Development Economics*, 1(2): 242-271.

Ruel M.T., Garrett J.L., Morris S.S., Maxwell D., Oshaug O., Engle P., Menon P., Slack A., Haddad L. (1998). "Urban challenges to food and nutrition security: A review of food security, health, and care giving in the cities". *Food Consumption and Nutrition Division Discussion Paper No 51*, International Food Policy Research Institute, Washington, D.C.

Ruel M.T., Haddad L., Garrett J.L. (1999). "Some urban facts of life: Implications for research and policy", *World Development*, 27(11): 1917-1938.

Ruel M.T., Haddad L., Garrett J.L. (1999). "Some urban facts of life: Implications for research and policy", *World Development*, 27(11): 1917-1938.

Ruel M.T., Menon P. (2002). "Creating a child feeding index using the demographic and health surveys: An example from Latin America". *Food Consumption and Nutrition Division Discussion Paper No. 130*, International Food Policy Research Institute, Washington DC.

Ruger J.P., Kim H.J. (2006). "Global health inequalities: an international comparison", *Journal of Epidemiology and Community Health*, 60(11): 928–936.

Ruzicka Lado T., Kane P. (1985). "Nutrition and child survival in South Asia." : 333-57.

Sakisaka K., Jimba M., Hanada K. (2010). "Changing poor mother's care-seeking behaviours in response to childhood illness: findings from a cross-sectional study in Granada, Nicaragua", *BMC International Health and Human Rights*, 10:10.

Sanfilippo M., de Neubourg C. Martorano B. (2012). "The Impact of Social Protection on Children: A Review of the Literature." Working Paper 2012-06, UNICEF, Florence.

Schellenberg J.A. (2003). "Inequities among the very poor: Health care for children in rural southern Tanzania". Ifakara Health Research and Development Center. Tanzania.

Schoenbaum M., Tulchinsky T.H., Abed Y. (1995). "Gender differences in nutritional status and feeding patterns among infants in the Gaza Strip." *American Journal of Public Health,* 85(7): 965-969.

Sen A. (1987). "Gender and cooperative conflicts". No. 1342. UNU Wider, Helsinki.

Setboonsarng, S. (2005). "Child Malnutrition as a Poverty Indicator: An Evaluation in the Context of Different Development Interventions in Indonesia". *Institute Discussion Paper*. No. 21. Asian Development Bank.

Sharma M., Sarangi B.L., Kanungo J., Sahoo S., Tripathy L., Patnaik A., Tewari J., Rath A.D. (2009). "Accelerating Malnutrition Reduction in Orissa". *IDS Bulletin*. 40(4): 78-85.

Shea K.M. (2007). "Global climate change and children's health". *Pediatrics*, 120, 1359–67.

Shekar M., Lee Y. (2006). "Mainstreaming nutrition in poverty reduction strategy papers: What does it take? A review of the early experience." *Health Nutrition and Population Discussion Paper*. The World Bank.

Shiva Kumar A.K. (2007). "*Why are child malnutrition levels not improving*?" Opinion- Leader Page Articles in The Hindu, Jun 23.

Sinha G., Peters D.H., Bollinger R.C. (2009). "Strategies for gender-equitable HIV services in rural India", *Health Policy and Planning*, 24(3): 197-208.

Skoufias E., Conroy H.V., Vinha K. (2011). The impacts of climate variability on welfare in rural Mexico. The World Bank, Poverty Reduction and Economic Management Network, Poverty Reduction and Equity Unit.

Skrondal A., Hesketh S.R. (2007). Multilevel and Longitudinal Modeling Using Stata. Statacorp LP.

Smith L.C., Haddad L. (2000). "Explaining Child Malnutrition in Developing Countries: A Cross-Country Analysis", Food Consumption and Nutrition Division Discussion Paper 60. International Food Policy Research Institute, Washington D.C.

Smith, L., Ruel, M.T., Ndiaye, A. (2005). "Why is child malnutrition lower in urban than in rural areas? Evidence from 36 developing countries", *World Development*, 33(8): 1285-1305.

Soeung S. C., *et al.* "Improving immunization coverage through budgeted microplans and sub-national performance agreements: early experience from Cambodia." *Asia Pacific Journal of Public Health*, 18(1): 29-38.

Som S., Pal M., Bharati P. (2007). "Role of individual and household level factors on stunting: A comparative study in three Indian states". *Annals of Human Biology*. 34(6): 632–646.

Sommerfelt E.A., Arnold F. (1998). "Undernutrition among boys and girls. Too young to die: Genes or gender". 133-153.

Sommerfelt E.A.. (1991). "Comparative analysis of the determinants of childrens nutritional status." [Unpublished]. Presented at the Demographic and Health Surveys World Conference Washington DC August 5-7 1991., 1991.

Sommerfelt, E.A., Stewart M.K. (1994). "Children's nutritional status."

Sonowal, C.J. (2010). "Factors affecting the nutritional health of tribal children in Maharashtra." *Ethno Med,* 4(1): 21-36.

Steinhardt L.C., Water H., Rao K.D., Naeem. A.J., Hansen. P., Peters D.H. (2009). "The effect of wealth status on care seeking and health expenditures in Afghanistan", *Health Policy and Planning*, 24(1): 1-17.

Strauss J., Thomas D. (1998). "Health, Nutrition, and Economic Development", *Journal of Economic Literature*, 36(2): 766-817.

Svedberg P. (2006). "Child malnutrition in shining India: A x-state empirical analysis". Institute for Economic Studies, Stockholm. Available at http:/ /www.bvsde.paho.org/bvsacd/cd56/svedberg-070906.pdf.

Svedberg P. (2007). "Child Malnutrition in India and China. 2020 focus brief on the world's poor and hungry people", International Food Policy Research Institute, Washington, DC.

Svedberg P. (2008). "Why Malnutrition in Shining India Persists". 4th Annual Conference on Economic Growth and Development, New Delhi.

Svedberg, P. (2000) "Poverty and Under-Nutrition: Theory, Measurement and Policy". Oxford University Press, Oxford. http://dx.doi.org/10.1093/ 0198292686.001.0001

Swaminathan M S. (2001). "Food security and sustainable development", *Current Science*, 81(8): 948-954.

Taguri A., Betilmal I., Mahmud S.M., Ahmed A.M., Goulet O., Galan P., Hercberg S. (2008) "Risk Factors for Stunting among Under-Fives in Libya". *Public Health Nutrition*, 12, 1141-1149. http://dx.doi.org/10.1017/ S1368980008003716

Tanner T., Mitchell T. (2008). "Entrenchment or enhancement: Could climate change adaptation help to reduce chronic poverty?" *IDS Bulletin*, 39(4): 6–15.

The United Nations Children's Fund. (1990). "Strategy for Improved Nutrition of Children and Women in Developing Countries".

The United Nations Children's Fund. (1998). "The State of the World's Children".

The World Bank. (2009). "Poverty and Climate Change Reducing the Vulnerability of the Poor through Adaptation".Washington DC.

The World Health Organization (2001). "Globalization, trade and public health: tools and training for national action", available at http://whqlibdoc.who.int/searo/2001/SEA_HSD_244.pdf

The World Health Organization. (1998). "Complementary feeding of young children in developing countries: a review of current scientific knowledge", available at http://whqlibdoc.who.int/hq/1998/WHO_NUT_98.1.pdf

The World Health Organization. (1999). "The world health report: making a difference.

Thomas D., Strauss J., Henriques M.H. (1990). "Child survival, height for age and household characteristics in Brazil", *Journal of Development Economics*, 33(2): 197–234.

Timaeus I.M., Lush L. (1995). "Intra-urban differentials in child health". *Health Transition Review*. 5:163–90.

Tinh, D.Q., Hang P.T. (2003). "Living with floods in Mekong river delta of Vietnam". Paper presented at the III World Water Forum- Poverty and Flood Theme. Available at http://www.adb.org/Documents/Events/2003/3WWF/Floods_Mekong.pdf.

Tipping G., Segall M. (1996). "Using a longitudinal illness record to study household health care decision-making in Rural communes of Viet Nam". *Health Policy and Planning*. 11(2):206-211.

United Nations International Children's Educational Fund. (2010). "Investing in nutrition for national growth and prosperity in Tanzania".

United Nations International Children's Fund. (2009). "Climate change and children in the Brasilian Amazon region".

Van Doorslaer E., Masseria C., Koolman X., & OECD Health Equity Research Group. (2006). "Inequalities in access to medical care by income in developed countries". *Canadian Medical Association Journal*, 174(2), 177-183.

Vella V., Tomkins A., Borghesi A., Migliori G.B., Adriko B.C., Crevatin E. (1992). "Determinants of child nutrition and mortality in north-west Uganda". *Bulletin of the World Health Organization*, 70(5): 637.

Victora C.G., Fall. C., Sachdev H., Adair L., Richter L., Hallal P., Martorell. R. (2008). Maternal and child undernutrition: Consequences for adult health and human capital. *The Lancet*, 371(9609), 340–357.

Victora C.G., Wagstaff A., Schellenberg J.A., Gwatkin D., Claeson M., Habicht J.P. (2003). "Applying an equity lens to child health and mortality: more of the same is not enough", *The Lancet*, 362(9379): 233–241.

Vijayaraghavan K., *et al*. (1990). "Effect of massive dose vitamin A on morbidity and mortality in Indian children." *The Lancet*. 336(8727): 1342-1345.

Visaria, L. (1987). "Sex differentials in nutritional status in a rural area of Gujarat state: an interim report."

Wagstaff A. (2000a). "Socio-economic inequalities in child mortality: comparisons across nine developing countries", *Bulletin of the World Health Organization*, 78(1): 19–29.

Wagstaff A. (2000b). "Caring more about the poor: inequality aversion, health inequalities, and health achievements", The World Bank, Washington DC.

Wagstaff A. (2002) "Poverty and Health Sector Inequalities". *Bulletin of the World Health Organization*, 80, 97-105.

Wagstaff A. (2003) Child Health on a Dollar a Day: Some Tentative Cross-Country Comparisons. *Social Science & Medicine*, 57, 1529-1538. http://dx.doi.org/10.1016/S0277-9536(02)00555-5

Wagstaff A. and van Doorslaer E. (2000). "Equity in Health Care Finance and Delivery". In: Culyer, A. and Newhouse, J.P., Eds., Handbook of Health Economics 1B, Elsevier Science, Amsterdam, 1803-1861. *http://dx.doi.org/10.1016/S1574-0064(00)80047-5*

Wagstaff A.,Van Doorslaer E. (2001). "What makes the personal income tax progressive? A comparative analysis for fifteen OECD countries." *International Tax and Public Finance*, 8(3): 299-316.

Wagstaff, A., Doorslaer, E., Watanabe, N. (2003). "On decomposing the causes of health sector inequalities with an application to malnutrition inequalities in Vietnam", *Journal of Econometrics*, 112(1): 207-223.

Walt G., Shiffman J., Schneider H., Murray S.F., Brugha R.,Gilson L. (2008). "Doing health policy analysis: methodological and conceptual reflections and challenges", *Health Policy and Planning*, 23(5):308-317.

West, Keith P., et al. (1991). "Efficacy of vitamin A in reducing preschool child mortality in Nepal." *The Lancet* 338(8759): 67-71.

Wolgemuth J.C., Latham M.C., Hall A., Chesher A., Crompton D.W. (1982). "Worker productivity and the nutritional status of Kenyan road construction laborers". *The American Journal of Clinical Nutrition*, 36(1), 68-78.

World Development Report. 1993: "Investing in health". The World Bank, Washington, DC.

Yambi O, Kavishe F.P. (1999). "Determinants of malnutrition, household food security, care and health", UNICEF ESARO, Nairobi, Kenia, paper prepared for BASIS (Broadening access and strengthening input market systems), (http://www.ies.wisc.edu/ltc/live/basissem 9911.pdf).

Yambi, O, Kavishe, F.P. (1999). "Determinants of malnutrition, household food security, care and health", UNICEF ESARO, Nairobi, Kenia, paper prepared for BASIS (Broadening access and strengthening input market systems), 13 The United Nations Children's Fund. Nairobi no date (http://www.ies.wisc.edu/ltc/live/basissem9911.pdf).

Zaman H. (1998). "Who Benefits and to What Extent? An Evaluation of BRAC's Micro-Credit Program". University of Sussex, Sussex.

Zaman H. (2000). "Assessing the Poverty and Vulnerability Impact of Micro-Credit in Bangladesh: A Case Study of BRAC". The World Bank, Washington DC.

Zeger S.L., Edelstein S.L. (1989). "Poisson regression with a surrogate X; an analysis of vitamin A and Indonesian children's mortality." *Applied Statistics,*: 309-318.

Zere E., McIntyre D. (2003). "Inequities in under-five child malnutrition in South Africa". *International Journal for Equity in Health*, 2(7): 1–10.

References Linked to This Book

Mukherjee, M., Mukherjee, A. (2014). Inclusive growth focus: Pattern of inequity in childhood nutritional achievement. *Challenges in Management and Information Technology (CMIT-2014)*. PP: 73-91, ISBN No: 978-81-8424-900-2, New Delhi, India.

Mukherjee, M., Mukherjee, A. (2014).Undernutrition poverty linkage: Analysis of literature with special focus on children. *Challenges in Management and Information Technology (CMIT-2014)*. PP: 92-109, ISBN No: 978-81-8424-900-2, New Delhi, India.

Mukherjee, M. (2015). Resilience-Vulnerability Dynamics and Under-nutrition in the Sundarbans Delta Region in India: Impacts, consequences and suggested responses. *International Journal of Development Research,*5(1): 3173-3183.

Mukherjee, M. (2015). Childhood under-Nutrition and SES Gradient in India – Myth or Reality. *Science Journal of Public Health.* 3(1): 119-137. doi: 10.11648/j.sjph.20150301.31

Mukherjee, M. (2016). Climatic Shock and Health Demand-Supply Nexus in the Sundarbans Delta Region in India. *Climate Change*, 2(5), 11-24.

Subject Index

G

H

I

L

M

N

P